HEALTH PROMOTION

THE BASICS

Health Promotion: The Basics introduces not only the fundamental theories and key concepts within this important area of health and social care, but translates these into practice for anyone working in the field.

The chapters are structured around the WHO's Ottawa Charter (1986) which underpins the discipline, and cover a comprehensive range of topics. From developing personal skills to understanding government policy, the book looks at health promotion on both an individual and a societal level. It spotlights key topic areas from behaviour change to climate change, as well as exploring how where we live impacts our health, and features practical examples for integrating health promotion into existing service provision and through community action.

Including case studies throughout, and further reading for those wishing to explore specific topics, this is the perfect introduction to what health promotion means and how it can improve everyday lives.

Nova Corcoran, PhD, is Senior Lecturer and Course Leader of the MSc Public Health at the University of South Wales, UK.

THE BASICS SERIES

The Basics is a highly successful series of accessible guidebooks which provide an overview of the fundamental principles of a subject area in a jargon-free and undaunting format.

Intended for students approaching a subject for the first time, the books both introduce the essentials of a subject and provide an ideal springboard for further study. With over 50 titles spanning subjects from artificial intelligence (AI) to women's studies, *The Basics* are an ideal starting point for students seeking to understand a subject area.

Each text comes with recommendations for further study and gradually introduces the complexities and nuances within a subject.

ECONOMICS (FOURTH EDITION)
Tony Cleaver

ELT
Michael McCarthy and Steve Walsh

SOLUTION-FOCUSED THERAPY
Yvonne Dolan

ACTING (THIRD EDITION)
Bella Merlin

BUSINESS ANTHROPOLOGY
Timothy de Waal Malefyt

EATING DISORDERS
Elizabeth McNaught, Janet Treasure, and Jess Griffiths

TRUTH
Jc Beall and Ben Middleton

PERCEPTION
Bence Nanay

For a full list of titles in this series, please visit
www.routledge.com/The-Basics/book-series/B

HEALTH PROMOTION

THE BASICS

Nova Corcoran

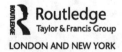

Routledge
Taylor & Francis Group

LONDON AND NEW YORK

Designed cover image: ©Getty

First published 2024
by Routledge
4 Park Square, Milton Park, Abingdon, Oxon OX14 4RN

and by Routledge
605 Third Avenue, New York, NY 10158

Routledge is an imprint of the Taylor & Francis Group, an informa business

British Library Cataloguing-in-Publication Data
A catalogue record for this book is available from the British Library

ISBN: 978-1-032-61165-5 (hbk)
ISBN: 978-1-032-20538-0 (pbk)
ISBN: 978-1-003-46232-3 (ebk)

DOI: 10.4324/9781003462323

Typeset in Bembo
by MPS Limited, Dehradun

CONTENTS

FIGURES

ACKNOWLEDGEMENTS

Thank you to Ben, Ostyn and Huxley who listened to me read and talk about this book for many months.

This book has been written for all my students, past and present, for whom I will always be their 'Dr Nova'.

WELCOME TO HEALTH PROMOTION

The basics

If health promotion was an item on a supermarket shelf, it would be resigned to the sale section at the back of the store. It would sit alongside other items that are still useful but no longer fashionable. But as every savvy shopper knows, with a little time and patience, the back of the store is where the bargains are to be found. And health promotion is exactly that; 'a bargain'. It is good value for money, and not only that, it makes all the other items nearby cheaper as well, rather like a buy-one-get-one-free (BOGOF). If you invest in health promotion, you save money on medical treatments like pharmaceutical drugs. If you invest in health promotion you save money in your economy as your workforces are healthier. If you invest in health promotion your population is healthier and happier. If you invest in health promotion you are quite simply 'getting a bargain'.

As fashions come and go, so too does the popularity of health promotion. Health issues, and how we respond to them change over time. Health is influenced by areas such as politics, economics and technology. Health needs differ across time and space. Accordingly, health promotion experiences the same variations. For example, cigarettes were once endorsed by doctors before studies showed

DOI: 10.4324/9781003462323-1

they caused cancer. Would the average person on the street today say that smoking is recommended for good health?

In early 2023 the World Health Organization (WHO) outlined the five health priorities for the next five years; see https://www. youtube.com/watch?v=Zs8flMvhCM4. Priority number one is 'promoting health' to address the root causes of disease. This shows us the value that global organisations place on health promotion. In the United Kingdom (UK), the trend for health promotion has actually decreased and although university courses still exist in health promotion, they tend to be bundled together with Public Health. However, if we look at other countries around the world high value is still placed on health promotion, and its sisters 'Health Education' and 'Health Communication'. Warwick-Booth et al. (2018) draw attention to places such as Ghana and Zambia where health promotion is still prized and supported.

You only need to tune into the news to see the significance of health in our everyday lives. Climate change, Covid-19 (coronavirus), conflict and the rising cost of living are frequent topics. It is becoming more important than ever that we maximise the potential of health promotion and bring it back into everything we do. As you will find out in this book, the discipline of health promotion is wide-ranging, and you don't need to work in health to do health promotion. You just need you, a desire to change things, and this book.

This book is designed to do two things. Firstly, I want to increase your knowledge of health promotion theory and practice. This is important for understanding why we do things the way we do. The second purpose is to introduce you to a wide range of health promotion skills through thinking exercises and activities that you can do wherever you are reading this book.

Ultimately health promotion is a practical, skills-based discipline that works with people. I have tried to imagine you in one of my classrooms where I teach not just health promotion theory, but the art of health promotion. Everyone has the potential to be a health promoter who can act, respond and inspire change. As I cannot bring you into my classroom, I have tried to bring the classroom to you. The examples and activities I give you in this book are from inside and outside the UK. To get the most out of this book you should consider 'adopting' a UK nation (England, Northern Ireland,

Scotland or Wales) and a country outside the UK so you can explore health promotion in different contexts.

Most of the time all you will need is a pencil and paper. If you don't have paper write notes in your copy of this book (unless it belongs to a library!). Sometimes you will need access to the internet to follow up on links or look at specific resources. Ultimately, I hope by reading this book you will have a better understanding of what health promotion is, and you will be inspired to be part of the future of health promotion.

REFERENCE

Warwick-Booth, L., Cross, R., Woodall, J., Bagnall, A.-M., & South, J. (2018). Health promotion education in changing and challenging times: Reflections from England. *Health Education Journal*, 78(6), 692–704. 10.1177/001789691 8784072.

1

THE FIELD OF HEALTH PROMOTION

DOI: 10.4324/9781003462323-2

- Wider reading
- Summary

OVERVIEW

Health promotion is quite simply what those two words suggest; it is the promotion of health. The word 'promotion' has many meanings including to support or encourage, to publicise or advertise, or to raise someone. Health promotion tries to do all of these things, as it supports people to change behaviours and improve their health. The word 'Health' is complex as you will see shortly, but if you take the meaning of health historically, it has been used to mean 'to heal', 'salvation', 'prosperity', 'welfare' and 'wholeness'. Health is important to us, and we may need to be 'healed' to get back to our 'whole' selves. We might even wish 'good health' on others. By promoting health, we are usually trying to make health better for people so they can live to their full potential. We will first start by defining health before we then look in more detail at what health promotion is.

WHAT IS HEALTH?

Practitioner skills activity 1a: What is health?

What does it mean to be healthy? How would you define health? If someone asked you if you were healthy, what would you say? Do you think other people think about health the same way you do?

A single definition of health does not exist as health is 'contested'. This means that what health is, is still argued about or debated. There is no one agreed definition of what health is, or how to measure it. What most people agree on is that health is important and that money should be used to secure good health. In the UK, the National Health Service (NHS) has provided universal healthcare (UHC) for over 75 years and is free for all at the point of access (Friebel et al., 2018). You can read more on UHC in Chapter 6 'Building healthy public policy'. The NHS is important to most UK citizens as illustrated in one of the stay-at-home messages during the first wave of Covid-19 to 'stay at home, protect the NHS' (Department of Health and Social Care, 2021). Communities even applauded frontline staff in weekly claps for 10 weeks from March 2020.

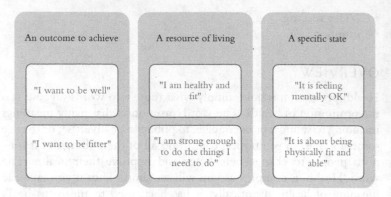

Figure 1.1 Different concepts of health.

Figure 1.1 shows the different ways people think about health. Sometimes it is an outcome that people want to achieve as most people would agree they want 'good health'. Other people think of health as a resource that lets them do what they want to do. It can also be a state, such as 'being in' good mental health. 'Medical' (sometimes called biomedical) definitions of health focus on the absence of disease or illness. A 'social' definition of health is much broader or 'holistic' and it can include mental health, spiritual health, physical health or well-being. In health promotion, the most commonly referred to definition of health comes from the World Health Organization (WHO), where health is defined as 'a state of complete physical, mental and social well-being and not merely the absence of disease or infirmity (World Health Organization, 1948). The Ottawa Charter for Health Promotion (World Health Organization, 1986) suggests health is a 'resource' for living as well as 'a state of complete physical, mental and social well-being including the ability of a person to meet their needs, realise aspirations and cope with their environment.

'The Adelaide Statement on Health in All Policies' (World Health Organization, 2010) summarises the importance of good health clearly by stating that 'good health enhances the quality of life, improves workforce productivity, increases learning capacity, strengthens families and communities, supports sustainable habitats and environments, and contributes to security, poverty reduction and social inclusion' (p.2). Health is, therefore, a resource for living that is highly desirable, and that has the potential to improve the quality and quantity of our lives.

WHAT IS HEALTH PROMOTION?

You have probably done something to promote your health, or the health of someone else, without even realising that you were doing health promotion. If you have ever resolved to do more exercise, change what you eat, quit smoking, or cut down on alcohol then you have done 'health promotion' on yourself. This is what is meant by the phrase 'taking responsibility for your health'. Perhaps you told someone else to try these things or supported them when they tried to change their behaviour. You might have been the recipient of health promotion for example being screened for cancer or receiving a vaccination. You might have had health promotion at school or work, for example, wellness days, sexual health education or mental health support. You might have read, watched, or listened to messages about health through mass media or information technology and you may be able to recall these messages. See the example below about Coronavirus (Covid-19) and mass media.

Health promotion in practice example: Coronavirus (Covid-19) mass media messages.

Many countries received mass media messages about Covid-19 in early 2020. These messages were designed to tell us about the rules and restrictions designed to protect people from Covid-19. Given how Covid-19 has pervaded our daily lives globally, most people will be able to recall some of the protective health messages given to the general public such as wearing a face covering, social distancing, or regular hand washing.

Health promotion is not just about giving people health information. Thinking of health promotion in this way assumes that the act of promoting or improving health is just about telling people what to do, or 'educating people'. Health promotion is much more than this. There are many ways to promote health that we do not typically think of as health promotion. Volunteering regularly for a local group or organisation can improve both your own and others' health. Reducing your household carbon footprint by walking to work can improve your health and protect the planet. Using your skills to support others to help them manage their health, for example, as a carer, helps improve the health of others. Campaigning for action about issues that you feel are unfair or unjust is also a type of health promotion action. These are not always the examples that come to mind when we think of health promotion, but they are all championing the same goal; to improve the health and well-being of you, your family, your community or wider society.

Health promotion is about preventing disease before it happens, rather than curing a disease. The phrase '*an ounce of prevention is worth a pound of cure*' attributed to Franklin (1735) was originally written in the context of how to protect towns from fire, but it encapsulates the way we think of health promotion practice today. If we promote health and prevent morbidity (sickness) and death (mortality), this is better than waiting for people to become unwell and then trying to 'cure them'. Most disease outcomes are better when diseases are either prevented or identified early, for example, cancers can be easier to treat when they are found in their earlier stages.

Practitioner skills activity 1b: Prevention or cure?
Think about your own country. What do you think you would make the priority in terms of diseases you could prevent? Would it cost more to prevent these diseases or cure these diseases?

There are also infections without a cure like HIV, where treatment is complex, for example, multidrug-resistant TB, or where the disease and its treatments may impact negatively the quality of life, such as chemotherapy for cancer. This does not mean that medicine and curative advances in this area are not important to health. The Office of National Statistics (2017) says in its analysis of deaths in the last 100 years that both medical science and better sanitation, hygiene, and nutrition are the main factors in why we live longer today than 100 years ago. Numerous medical and scientific advances could be cited as important to improving the health of populations. They include the discovery of antibiotics or insulin and screening tests for sexually transmitted infections (STIs) or cancers.

THE ORIGINS OF HEALTH PROMOTION

Health promotion has been around for a long time. We have just been calling it different things. Hippocrates, who lived over 2000 years ago, was one of the first people to be credited with referring to disease as being caused by environmental factors and the way we live our lives, such as our diet (Porter, 1999). Health Promoters today advocate for healthy environments such as those free from pollution along with healthy lifestyle behaviours such as eating a healthy diet.

Madsen (2017) suggests that health promotion became more established in the 19th century (the 1800s) as literacy in the general population increased, definitions of health changed to include individual behaviours and health education materials were published. In the UK, this may also have coincided with the Industrial Revolution, for example, Gems (2021) suggests that the development of new types of sport and recreational activities such as swimming, came from better income, transport, and eventually better working conditions and consequently more leisure time.

Examples of what we recognise as health promotion became most visible in the UK from the early 1900s. For example, by the 1920s there was increased emphasis in schools on playground-based activity linked to new laws in education that saw physical education (PE) as a form of preventive medicine and good for children's health (Welshman, 1998). In the 1930s the 'Women's League of Health and Beauty' was a popular women's fitness organisation across the UK and was a means of empowering women to take charge of their health (Heffernan, 2019). One of the first examples of a 'healthy living centre' is the Peckham Experiment in London opened in 1935. This was a 'pioneer health centre' set up for families who lived within one mile of the centre to improve health through health checks and recreational activities for a small user fee (Socialist Health Association, 2022).

DEFINING HEALTH PROMOTION

As many authors have noted, the term 'health promotion' is relatively new and 'health education' or 'health communication' are sometimes more commonly used terms. More recently the term 'public health' has also been used instead of health promotion in the UK, but they were originally two separate areas, and using public health in this way is not true to the origins of health promotion. There is no agreed definition of health promotion but many of the ways people define health promotion are quite similar. The 'Ottawa Charter for Health

Promotion' is probably the first to define health promotion as we see it today. It states health promotion is the 'process of enabling people to increase control over and to improve their health' (World Health Organization, 1986). This definition captures the idea that health promotion supports people through actions to improve their health.

Practitioner skills activity 1c: What is health promotion?

Which of the activities in the list do you think are health promotion activities?

- *Using posters and leaflets to encourage individuals to be physically active.*
- *Campaigning for an increased tax on tobacco products.*
- *Running low-cost exercise classes for older people at local community centres.*
- *Teaching a curriculum of PSHE (personal, social, health and economic) education in a school.*
- *Providing a re-use, re-cycle and repair centre in the local community*

The National Institute of Clinical Excellence (NICE) is an organisation that provides evidence of best practices in healthcare. They refer to health promotion as 'giving people the information or resources they need to improve their health. As well as improving people's skills and capabilities, it can also involve changing the social and environmental conditions and systems that affect health' (National Institute of Clinical Excellence, 2022). This definition tells us more about the ways that health promotion can support people by giving information and helping to improve personal skills. Personal skills are things like increasing self-esteem or confidence. Chapter 2 'Developing personal skills' focuses on personal skills. This definition also highlights the environment and the conditions in which we live. This means the factors around us that influence health, for example, housing, jobs or transport. Chapter 4 'Creating supportive environments' discusses this more.

Green et al. (2019) include the concepts of 'health education' and 'healthy public policy' in their definition of health promotion. This echoes previous examples but also introduces us to the idea of 'healthy public policy'. Healthy public policies contribute to good health, such as laws to prevent discrimination like the Equality Act 2010 (Government Equalities Office, 2010), or banning the direct

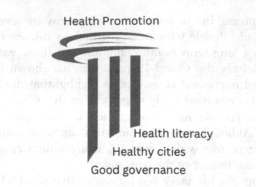

Health Promotion

Health literacy
Healthy cities
Good governance

Figure 1.2 The three pillars of health promotion.

and indirect advertising of tobacco to young people. Healthy public policy is the focus of Chapter 6 'Building healthy public policy'.

Finally, the 'Shanghai Declaration on Health Promotion' (World Health Organization, 2016) adds the notion of three pillars of health promotion; these are health literacy, good governance and healthy cities. Figure 1.2 shows the three pillars of health promotion.

- Health literacy is people's ability to understand and act on health information. This is covered in Chapter 2 'Developing personal skills'.
- Good governance is connected to health policy and means ensuring policies are created and implemented to ensure healthy choices are accessible to all. This is covered more in Chapter 6 'Building healthy public policy'.
- Over half the global population live in cities, and we need to be able to live and work in cities that promote health. Healthy cities reflect previous global public health documents on the importance of healthy settings. You can learn more about healthy settings in Chapter 4 'Creating supportive environments'.

HEALTH PROMOTION TODAY; CORONAVIRUS (COVID-19)

In 2019 the first reports of a new virus spreading rapidly across the world were circulating in the media. This virus became known as 'Covid-19'. Covid-19 is caused by a coronavirus and causes fever or cough symptoms, but in some cases, symptoms are severe and can result in death. People who are at the highest risk are older, those living with a long-term health condition and those with low immunity. Globally the Covid-19 pandemic has shown us how interconnected our world is, as well as highlighting the inequalities between who was most likely to get sick or die. Covid-19 disrupts systems that provide food, energy, services and goods including healthcare. Although it appears the worst times are ending and we are learning to live with Covid-19, many countries are still experiencing the impact of the pandemic.

Aside from the mortality and morbidity that Covid-19 infection causes, there are also other consequences of Covid-19. Research shows that school closures make worse existing inequalities in student attainment and engagement in learning which widen the learning gap between the richest and poorest pupils (Darmody et al., 2021). The World Economic Forum (2021) highlights that during the worst parts of the pandemic, 1.5 billion students in 188 countries were unable to attend school which may have lasting consequences on young people. In some countries, particularly low and middle-income countries, the most vulnerable are more likely to drop out of school, and literacy skills show a large decrease when children are out of school for one year or more.

Data from the Office of National Statistics in the UK suggest that around 1 in 25 adults report long Covid, which is illness, 12 to 20 weeks after the first Covid-19 infection (Office of National Statistics, 2023). This is a previously unknown condition. Research by Tene et al. (2023) shows that long Covid is associated with the increased use of healthcare services and that a wide range of health services are needed to support people in their long Covid recovery.

HEALTH PROMOTION TODAY; THE RISING COST OF LIVING

The 'cost of living' is the amount of money that people pay to maintain a good quality of life and includes their spending on areas like housing, energy and food. The money that we have to spend to support our quality of life is called 'disposable income'. This is the amount of income we have after tax. The cost of living has risen dramatically in many countries in the last two years. In the UK the cost of living as of March 2023 was the highest it has been for 41 years (Francis–Devine et al., 2023). This is largely driven by big increases in the cost of food, energy, housing and fuel (Public Health Wales, 2022).

When prices rise with inflation, and people's income does not rise at the same rate, this has major health consequences if people are unable to afford what they need, for example, shelter, food or heat. At the end of 2022, Public Health Scotland published a Health Impact Assessment (HIA) on the rising cost of living. Chapter 6 'Building healthy public policy' has more on HIAs. It identifies many negative impacts of increased costs including debt, food insecurity, fuel poverty, homelessness, mental distress, crime and family violence and reduced social interaction (Public Health Scotland, 2022). Those at highest risk are those who are already living in poverty or who are earning a low income, as well as specific population groups such as those living in rural communities, people who are renting, lone parents and unemployed people (Public Health Wales, 2022). See also the later section on poverty in this chapter.

Practitioner skills activity 1d: Children and the rising cost of living.

Children in low-income households are likely to experience negative impacts from the rising cost of living. Give examples of how children's health might be impacted by the rising cost of living in your country. What do you think could be realistically done to support children in low-income households?

HEALTH PROMOTION TODAY; CONFLICT

Conflict is bad for health in any form. It causes death and disability and destroys communities and livelihoods. It has devastating consequences for people who live in conflict areas and for those who are forced to migrate from their homes. It stops progress on global goals such as the Sustainable Development Goals (SDGs) (see the next section for more on the SDGs). For example, challenges such as food and water shortages, reduced agriculture production, increased unemployment, destruction of infrastructures such as medical facilities and schools, and increased physical and mental harm significantly hinder SDG achievement (Pereira et al., 2022). At any one time, there is conflict happening in countries across the world, from small-scale rioting to large-scale warfare. The International Monetary Fund (IMF) (International Monetary Fund, 2022) estimates just under 1 billion people live in a fragile or conflict state. 'Fragile' refers to a weak country that is at risk of conflict due to limited capacity, lack of resources, unstable institutions like banks or businesses and political instability.

The most recent example of how conflict can have global impacts is the Russia–Ukraine conflict (2022 to present). The conflict has destroyed infrastructures and caused civilian deaths. The United Nations Refugee Agency estimates as of January 2023 there are around 8 million refugees across Europe, and in Ukraine, there are more than 5 million people displaced and 17.6 million people in need of humanitarian assistance (UNHCR, 2023). Outside the UK the conflict has increased global food and energy prices from a combination of country sanctions and supply chain disruption (Jagtap et al., 2022). These are the rules that are placed on countries such as Russia to limit trade, as well as the difficulties in trading that accompany conflict such as the inability to farm foods or sell goods. This results in competition for fewer resources such as oil, which pushes up prices. Chapter 4 'Creating supportive environments' discusses the impact on food environments. Russia–Ukraine is a rapidly changing situation, and for updates about the conflict see the resources at the end of the chapter.

HEALTH PROMOTION TODAY; CLIMATE CHANGE

Climate change refers to the process of global warming which is caused by increased amounts of greenhouse gases in the Earth's atmosphere. Greenhouse gases come from fossil fuels like oil and gas that we burn. The build-up of these gases causes a warming effect which we call climate change. The consequences of this are rising sea levels, more extreme weather, and changes to our planet's biodiversity such as plants and animals.

Climate change affects everyone, and it is now the biggest challenge facing our world. The WHO predicts between 2030 and 2050 approximately 250,000 additional deaths will occur through malnutrition, malaria, diarrhoea and heat stress linked to climate change

(World Health Organization, 2023). Those who are the most vulnerable experience the negative impacts of climate change the most. Extreme heat for example is a consequence of climate change. It is associated with increased morbidity and mortality, adverse impacts on pregnancy outcomes, negative effects on mental health and reduced productivity (Ebi et al., 2021). You can read more about heat and health in the Lancet series at https://www.thelancet.com/series/heat-and-health.

Health promotion has to support efforts to reduce climate change, prevent harm, and protect those most at risk. In addition, health promotion programmes and interventions should carry a low-carbon footprint, meaning they are sustainable and try and use low-carbon solutions. Climate change is discussed in many examples throughout this book.

Practitioner skills activity 1e: What are the challenges facing health?

What do you think are the challenges facing health in your country? Which populations do you think these challenges impact the most?

HEALTH PROMOTION TODAY; CHANGING DISEASE PATTERNS

Globally, the most common causes of death are now non-communicable diseases (meaning non-infectious diseases or 'chronic' diseases). Health promotion work in high-income countries predominately focuses on non-communicable diseases. Many risk factors for non-communicable diseases are linked to behaviour, this is why most people think health promotion is about changing lifestyles. However, non-communicable disease risks also come from our living and working conditions. For example, ischaemic heart disease (IHD) accounts for the most global deaths (approximately 16%) (World Health Organization, 2020). Mortality from IHD is linked to access to health services and economic growth, as well as risk factors such as high body mass index (BMI), diabetes mellitus and tobacco consumption (Nowbar et al. 2019). Health promotion action to reduce IHD and other communicable diseases needs a combination of approaches from supporting people with medication adherence to advocating for taxation on tobacco sales and promoting policies that support fair access to healthcare.

In low-income countries, disease patterns are different with six of the top ten causes of death being communicable diseases (World Health Organization, 2020). The leading cause of death in low-income countries is neonatal conditions. Goldenberg et al. (2018) state that the three main causes of neonatal mortality are asphyxia, infections such as sepsis and prematurity which can result in complications as babies are born too early. This is followed by lower respiratory infections such as pneumonia. In third place is IHD. This shows that lower-income countries are presented with the double challenge of dealing with both communicable and non-communicable diseases. As with IHD, reducing the leading causes of death in low-income countries is connected to improving living and working conditions such as reducing poverty and unemployment, promoting political stability, and increasing access to resources and services such as clean water, sanitation and healthcare. Chapter 6 'Building healthy public policy' discusses universal healthcare which is also vital.

SUSTAINABLE DEVELOPMENT GOALS

The Sustainable Development Goals (SDGs) are 17 global goals to be achieved by 2030 that aim to support humans to live to their full potential in a healthy environment. Adopted in 2015 and signed by 194 countries, each goal has targets and ways of measuring the targets through 'indicators'. We will be covering many examples of the goals throughout this book.

Globally, the SDGs dictate health promotion priorities in many countries. They include a focus on no poverty, zero hunger, gender equality, clean water and sanitation, reducing inequalities, sustainable cities and climate action. The 17 goals can be seen in Figure 1.3. The practitioner skills activity 1f encourages you to explore these more.

Practitioner skills activity 1f: Sustainable Development Goals (SDGs)
Look at the 17 SDGs at this link https://sdgs.un.org/goals. *Explore the resources available under 'topics' for areas of interest. For example:*
Water and sanitation https://sdgs.un.org/topics/water-and-sanitation.
Climate action https://sdgs.un.org/topics/climate-action-synergies.
Transport https://sdgs.un.org/topics/sustainable-transport.
Look up your country's progress on the SDGs on the dashboard at https://dashboards.sdgindex.org/profiles.

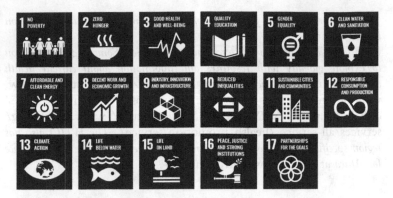

Figure 1.3 The 17 sustainable development goal icons.

HEALTH PROMOTION TOPICS

Every country and region is different when it comes to deciding the remit of health promotion. Today's health promoters are working towards a variety of local and global goals, which include the SDGs and national policies. More on national policies is in Chapter 6 'Building healthy public policy'.

Practitioner skills activity 1g: What is happening in your country?

What are the priorities for your country, region or locality? Use a search engine on the internet to locate your main Government health organisation, such as a Ministry of Health. Search for 'health promotion' or 'health education' on their website. What sort of Health promotion topics are given? Local councils and health care providers may also have information.

Examples of popular areas considered to be part of the health promotion remit can be found on country and regional area websites. The Department of Health (Northern Ireland) Health Promotion page (Department of Health (NI), 2022) has topics that include breastfeeding, food hygiene, obesity prevention, sexual health promotion, skin cancer prevention, substance use, suicide prevention and tobacco control. A look at other countries may reveal different priorities. For example, in Canada, topics include injury prevention, physical activity, family violence prevention and healthy pregnancy alongside population health programmes such as seniors' health, child health and rural health (Government of Canada, 2022).

Health promotion in practice example: Websites with health promotion topics.

Different countries have different health priorities. Some examples for you to explore globally with resources and information about current health campaigns include: *VicHealth in Victoria, Australia* https://www.vichealth.vic.gov.au/, *New York City* https://www.nyc.gov/site/doh/index.page, *NHS Fife in Scotland* https://www.nhsfife.org/services/all-services/health-promotion-service/, *The WHO also has region-specific Health Promotion information, for example, the regional office for Africa at* https://www.afro.who.int/.

THE SOCIAL DETERMINANTS OF HEALTH

The Jakarta Declaration on 'Leading Health Promotion into the 21st Century' (World Health Organization, 1997) states that health promotion can develop and change lifestyles and impact the social, economic and environmental conditions that determine health. The WHO and the United Nations both acknowledge that health is created by the conditions in which we live, work and play. These are called the social determinants of health.

Figure 1.4 shows some of the social determinants of health. It shows:

- **Individual determinants:** These include demographics like age, gender, ethnicity, disability, sexuality and our behaviours such as physical activity, diet, tobacco, alcohol, and sleep.
- **Community determinants:** These include social networks like friends, relationships, groups we belong to, community safety, schools, workplaces, housing, transport and access to services.
- **Structural determinants:** These include wider determinants such as economic growth, political stability, healthcare provision, peace, justice, spatial planning, climate and geography.

Several authors try and show the social determinants of health in a diagram format. The most commonly used in the UK is the Dahlgren and Whitehead 'Rainbow Model (Dahlgren & Whitehead, 1991), which was revised in 2021 (Dahlgren & Whitehead, 2021) to include a broader focus on policy. You can see this model and a range of other

Figure 1.4 The social determinants of health.

social determinants of health models here https://www.ncbi.nlm.nih.gov/books/NBK221240/. There have also been suggestions for modifications to existing social determinants of health models, for example Jahnel et al. (2022) propose the inclusion of digital technology within social determinants of health models, as when many models were designed the 'digital age' was little considered and post-covid-19 digital literacy has become more important. You can see this at https://www.ncbi.nlm.nih.gov/pmc/articles/PMC9530552/. Chapter 2 'Developing personal skills' also has a section on digital literacy.

Practitioner skills activity 1h: Social determinants of health.
Have a look at one of the social determinants of health models using the links above. Do they include all determinants that you think influence

health? If you created a social determinant of health model what would it look like? Which wider social determinants do you think have the most important influence on health? The Centre for Disease Control (CDC) (USA) has a video on the social determinants of health that you can watch at https://www.youtube.com/watch?v=u_IoBt7Nicw&t=2s.

POVERTY

Nearly half of the world's population live in poverty. People living in poverty face challenges obtaining the essentials to meet their basic needs like food, shelter and healthcare. In the UK, 13.4 million people live in poverty and just over half of these are working-age adults (Joseph Rowntree Foundation, 2023). Poverty is bad for health and it stops people from living to their full potential. Those living on low incomes are more likely to have poor mental health and low levels of well-being (Thomson et al., 2022) as well as poorer physical health.

Households who live in poverty are more likely to live in areas of high deprivation. 'Deprivation' means that areas may not have things essential to life like good quality housing and safe streets. This impacts different groups of people in different ways, for example, children may have fewer safe places to play and lower-quality schools. This then has an impact on their physical and mental health through lack of outdoor play, along with their educational attainment through poorer quality schooling.

Here are some examples of how poverty can affect health:

- Poor physical health from lack of heat, food, health care or shelter.
- Poor mental health such as stress, anxiety, depression or low self-esteem.
- Poor social health through the inability to participate in employment, recreational activities or social events and occasions.

The cost of living is rising dramatically in many countries, including the UK. This means that people who are already on low incomes are further vulnerable to the negative impacts of rising costs. Low-income households spend a larger proportion than average on energy and food, so are more affected by price increases (Francis-Devine et al., 2023). This means those who are the worst off are impacted the most by increases in the cost of living.

HEALTH FOR ALL

Despite one of the goals of the WHO being 'health for all', along with a focus on 'health as a human right', health is not equal. Some people have better health than others. Take the example of where you live. Globally life expectancy in some countries is much higher than in other countries. Our World in Data at https://ourworldindata.org/ says that:

- Life expectancy for the world is around 72 years.
- Life expectancy in Japan is around 85 years.
- Life expectancy for the Central African Republic is around 53 years.

There are also differences between groups of people within countries. For example, in the UK life expectancy is around 79 years for males and 82.9 years for females, showing a gender difference. There are also geographical differences between places, for example, England has a higher life expectancy than Scotland (Office of National Statistics, 2021). There are even differences within local areas. In London, life expectancy varies by up to ten years across London boroughs (Trust For London, 2022). There are more life expectancy resources at the end of the chapter.

If we look at 'healthy life expectancy' (which is the number of years you can expect to live in good health) we find similar differences. Those who live in areas of the highest deprivation can expect to live fewer years in good health than those in the least deprived areas. In Scotland for example, there can be differences in more than 20 years of life lived in good health across different places (Scottish Government, 2018). People who live in the most deprived communities are expected to spend more of their lives in poorer health and have a shorter life than those who live in the least deprived areas. This is simply not fair, and health promoters have a significant role to play in working to reduce health inequalities between and within populations. The World Health Organization has a 'Health for All' film festival which chooses a wide range of films to showcase around this theme. You can see these at https://www.who.int/initiatives/health-for-all-film-festival.

Practitioner skills activity 1i: Why is health unequal?
Use a search engine to look up two cities in the same county. For example, Aberdeen and Glasgow in Scotland, or Bristol and Liverpool in England. There are differences in life expectancy and healthy life expectancy in these cities even though they are in the same country. Why do you think there are differences? Think about which social determinants of health might cause these differences.

Explore the visual differences in health across the USA using the health map at https://vizhub.healthdata.org/subnational/usa *which shows differences across the country and states in life expectancy, mortality and risk factors such as diabetes and hypertension.*

HEALTH INEQUALITIES

Health is unequal. The 'Health for all' section previously highlighted differences between people and the places they live. There are also disparities in health by gender, ethnicity, sexuality, and disability, as well as across different disease conditions. These differ in different countries. For example, in the UK, although women live longer than men, women have been found to experience poorer healthcare outcomes than men, which is the reverse of many other countries (Winchester, 2021). Some countries also experience differences in ethnicity. For example, in the USA, there are consistent inequalities between different racial and ethnic groups, with people of colour experiencing worse social and economic conditions that influence health negatively (Hill, 2023). Data also shows that people living with a disability have poorer health outcomes than those without (Office of National Statistics, 2022). In many countries, people living with a disability are excluded from education and employment opportunities, and face barriers such as a lack of transport or non-existent disability-friendly services (Swenor, 2021).

Practitioner skills activity 1j: Health inequalities.
Choose either gender, ethnicity, sexuality or disability. Consider how health could be unequal in your country between population groups, for

example, different genders or sexualities. What differences might your chosen population group experience in areas like access to education, finance, healthcare or employment?

Inequalities are unfair and unjust. Health inequalities are influenced by the social determinants of health. Unequal access to resources such as housing or employment contributes to health inequalities. For example, across Europe, data shows that no matter how health is measured, those who have the lowest levels of education are more likely to be in poorer health, and people with less income are less likely to access healthcare (OECD, 2019).

In the UK, health inequalities appear to be worsening. For example, in Scotland, The Health Foundation (2023) shows how inequalities are getting worse for the most deprived communities, with trends in child health and young and mid-aged male health being of particular concern. Read more at https://www.health.org.uk/publications/leave-no-one-behind. The differences between health across population groups are not randomly distributed. Data consistently shows that those who are living in the most deprived areas, or who have the lowest levels of income have poorer health than those in the most affluent areas with the highest levels of income. This is not specific to the UK. Other countries show similar trends, for example in Australia death, disease and disability are higher in those with lower socio-economic status (Australian Institute of Health and Welfare, 2023).

The Health Foundation have a UK evidence-based resource that shows how determinants like work, housing, transport and income influence health and well-being (The Health Foundation, 2022). Take the determinant 'education' as an example. People with better education are more likely to have higher-quality jobs, higher incomes and good access to health care and they are more likely to understand and act on health information (McDaniel et al., 2017). The example of education shows us that determinants are interrelated and influence health in different ways. An example of how housing impacts health is in the health promotion in practice example below. There are more resources on health inequalities at the end of the chapter.

Health promotion in practice example: Housing and Health.
Housing influences health. Housing quality such as the state of a property can impact health such as hazards causing accidents, or damp homes making

respiratory conditions worse. The ability to afford quality housing also impacts health as those on lower incomes are less able to afford good housing in a safe, attractive neighbourhood. Lack of shelter decreases life expectancy and contributes to poor mental and physical well-being along with barriers to healthcare and participation in society. Read more about housing in high-income countries like the UK at the Health Foundation Evidence Hub https://www.health.org.uk/evidence-hub/housing. *The WHO has housing and health guidance with practical ways to improve housing at* https://www.who.int/publications/i/item/9789241550376. Chapter 5 *'Reorientating health services' has more on homelessness.*

HEALTH EQUITY

Health equity is about things being fair. Making things equal does not always make things fair. Some people need more help than others to have good health. If we offer everyone the same thing, or we treat everyone the same, then we fail to recognise that some people need more help to be more equal. For example, imagine you are running a Fall Prevention exercise class. This class teaches people strength and balance exercises to help reduce their fall risk. In the class, some people might find the exercises too hard, and some may have difficulty learning new information or hearing the instructions. Others may have a physical disability or injury which stops them from doing some of the exercises. Even though we are offering everyone the same thing (making things equal), not everyone can participate which means we are not making things fair.

Health equity, along with similar concepts like 'social justice' is when we work to make things fair across all sectors of society. This can be across characteristics that people are discriminated against like age, gender and ethnicity as well as the social determinants of health such as access to quality housing or employment opportunities.

WHAT DOES A HEALTH PROMOTER DO?

A health promoter is someone who can 'advocate, enable and mediate change' (World Health Organization, 1986). This is what this book hopes you will be able to do by the time you have finished reading it! Health promoters need to know the right skills and tools for action. They are also able to change the wider environmental, policy, and societal context that facilitates or hinders change. Health promoters also understand the wide variety of issues that impact health and how they influence different people unequally. Health promoters work to make things fairer and more equal for people experiencing inequalities in health.

Most health promoters are passionate about making things better for others, particularly in groups who might be disadvantaged in some way. This is not just through education but through environmental change, or public policies that improve health. This means a health promoter advocates on behalf of those who may not have a voice and communicates innovative and evidence-based solutions through oral or written communication means. A health promoter has skills to support people who want to make a change, for themselves or their communities. A health promoter also tries to encourage health in all policies, or healthy public policies and ensures that organisations and settings take responsibility for improving the health of the people that they serve.

ADVOCATE, ENABLE, MEDIATE

The main ways that a health promoter works is to advocate, enable and mediate change. These are areas that were specified by the Ottawa Charter for Health Promotion. Figure 1.5 represents these three areas visually, and the corresponding explanation follows below.

Advocate means an action that tries to make conditions conducive to health. The determinants of health mentioned previously are part of this. This is not individual biological factors like gender or ethnicity, but our lifestyle such as whether we exercise or smoke, and the wider social determinants such as housing, schools and workplaces. Politics, economic and environmental conditions are also important to health. Advocating for decent living and working conditions is part of health promotion practice.

Health promotion in practice example: Advocacy via food banks in the UK. The Trussell Trust aims to stop UK hunger. It supports a network of food banks to provide emergency food and campaigns to end the need for food banks in the UK including lobbying Government for action to ensure

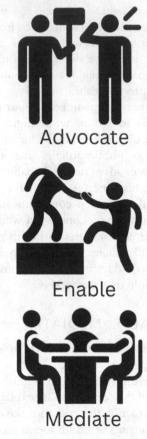

Figure 1.5 Advocate, enable and mediate change.

everyone has enough income to afford the essentials. You can find out more about their advocacy work at https://www.trusselltrust.org/get-involved/campaigns/.

Enable means action to help people achieve their full potential such as being able to read and understand health information or having the skills to make choices about health, as well as actioning these choices. It may be providing people with skills, resources, or conditions where change is supported and people feel more empowered to improve their health.

Health promotion in practice example: Enabling skills in Dementia Friends.
Dementia Friends is an Alzheimer's Society Initiative to change people's
perceptions of Dementia. A dementia friend is somebody who learns about
dementia so they can help people living within their community. You can
become a friend by using resources on the website or by joining an information
session held locally. To find out more visit https://www.dementiafriends.
org.uk/ *(England and Wales) or in Scotland* https://www.alzscot.org/
our-work/dementia-friendly-communities *which also has a dementia-*
friendly toolkit. Global Dementia Friends information can be found at
https://www.alzheimers.org.uk/about-us/policy-and-influencing/
global-dementia-friends-network. *Chapter 4 'Creating supportive en-*
vironments' also includes more on dementia-friendly communities.

Mediate means working to coordinate action between different
organisations that influence health. These might not be health organisations. Local governments, public organisations like schools,
voluntary organisations like charities, or private companies like
businesses can all impact health.

Health promotion in practice example: Mediating community safety in
England.
Community safety issues such as anti-social behaviour can negatively impact
health, and solutions need to involve multiple organisations and strategies.
Here are two examples of partnerships to improve community safety.

The London (England) Metropolitan Police run a 'walk and talks' scheme
for women over 18 living or working in London who would like to go for a
walk with an officer in their local area and discuss their views on women's
safety. Find out more here https://www.met.police.uk/police-forces/
metropolitan-police/areas/campaigns/2022/walk-and-talks/.

The Safer York (England) Partnership has examples of partners involved
in improving community safety and types of community safety projects
https://www.saferyorkpartnership.co.uk/.

Many health promotion campaigns focus on advocate, enable and
mediate together as the three areas overlap. The Zero Malaria
https://zeromalaria.org/ is a movement that aims to bring people
together to campaign for action from world leaders to reduce malaria. It started in Senegal (Africa) in 2014.

- The current campaign uses global ambassadors like athletes, singers, and actors combined with social media such as the film 'Turning up the pressure'. This is an example of 'advocate'.
- The campaign brings people together as one collective voice. One voice may not be very powerful by itself, but many voices are. The campaign urges individuals to take action together, for example in 2022 people were encouraged to engage with the website and 'draw the line' using a new language called the 'Muundo' designed by Nigerian artist Láolú Senbanjo. This is an example of 'mediate'.
- The Pan-Africa version of the campaign contains a wide range of resources to empower communities to take ownership of malaria action projects. Case studies, resources and toolkits are all available at https://zeromalaria.africa/resources. This is an example of 'enable'.

THE HEALTH PROMOTION ACTION AREAS

The Institute of Health Promotion and Health Education's position statement on health promotion (2021) states that health promotion is multifaceted, and includes building personal skills, creating healthy environments, ensuring health in all policies, reorientating health services, community action and an emphasis on healthy settings. These five areas are the core action areas of the Ottawa Charter for Health Promotion and form the basis for the chapters in this book. These are shown in Figure 1.6.

Figure 1.6 shows the action areas of the Ottawa Charter. Each chapter in this book will focus on each of the areas separately. The areas of the Ottawa Charter are all interconnected, and the charter is rarely used effectively when each area is only considered by itself. For example, SDG indicator 3.7 focuses on access to sexual and reproductive services including information, education and the integration of reproductive health into national strategies and programmes. Meeting this indicator needs more than one solution. Knowledge about Sexually transmitted infections (STIs) will not reduce STIs without the provision of free, and confidential contraception and treatment services ('building healthy public policy) in accessible community spaces ('reorientating health services'),

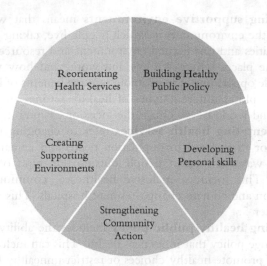

Figure 1.6 The Ottawa Charter for Health Promotion action areas (World Health Organization, 1986).

alongside formal and informal health education for young people ('developing personal skills'). However, to be able to create action like the STI example above, we need to learn about each area, how it works, and the practical ways the charter can be applied. Hence, for these purposes, the charter areas have been temporarily separated.

Developing personal skills is about the provision of health education and skills to help people to make healthy choices and exercise more control over their health. This chapter includes a focus on areas such as the ethics of health promotion, health communication, behaviour change, mass media, Information Technology (IT) and health literacy. This is the focus of Chapter 2.

Strengthening community action focuses on activities that support communities to improve their health and well-being. This includes using resources in communities to support health and well-being. This chapter includes a focus on core components of community activities using a wide range of examples from time banking and citizen science to housing developments and co-production. This is the focus of Chapter 3.

Creating supportive environments means that we need to consider the environments in which people live, taking care of our communities and our natural environment and resources. This includes the places where we live and work, and how we look at sustainable opportunities to promote positive benefits of health. The chapter explores different types of healthy settings such as cities, schools and workplaces. This is the focus of Chapter 4.

Reorientating health services refer to changing the health-care sector to respond to population needs and demands, and to consider ways to support people outside the remit of treatment services. This includes inclusive healthcare, community health promotion and climate change-resilient hospitals. This is the focus of Chapter 5.

Building healthy public policy includes the ability to change or challenge policy that influences health. This can include taxes or laws that promote healthy choices or restrict unhealthy behaviours. The chapter explores what policy is, how it is made and how we can predict its impact on health. This is the focus of Chapter 6.

HEALTH PROMOTION ACTION IN THIS BOOK

Each chapter has a variety of features to help support your learning. The 'Practitioner skills activities' are designed to increase your knowledge and skills in advocating, enabling and mediating for change. The 'Health promotion in practice examples' are case studies and scenarios from health promotion practice to help you see how what we talk about links with health promotion action. Many examples can't fit inside the pages of one book so I have given links to more information throughout. Whilst several of these examples might not call themselves 'health promotion' (remember the word is not fashionable in the UK) all the examples encapsulate the ethos of health promotion. Health promotion and the challenges it faces evolve, and whilst many of the principles stay the same the issues we face can change, as evidenced by the rising cost of living and Covid-19. This book aims to equip you with the basics but don't forget to also look at happening in the world outside your window to help you stay up to date. Each chapter has wider reading, listening and watching resources.

SUMMARY

You are now armed with a background in health and health promotion and how it has evolved to become the health promotion we use today. Now it is time to start your health promotion journey by learning about 'Developing personal skills' in the next chapter.

WIDER READING SUGGESTIONS

ONLINE

For more on the Social Determinants of Health look at models like the Barton and Grant (2010) Health map, https://www.wellbeingforlife.org.uk/sites/default/files/B&G%20determinants%20of%20h&w%20in%20our%20cities_0.pdf.

For more on the Social Determinants of Health in the context of England, see https://www.gov.uk/government/publications/health-profile-for-england-2018/chapter-6-wider-determinants-of-health#main-messages.

For more on life expectancy explore 'Our World in Data', https://ourworldindata.org/life-expectancy.

For more on health, inequalities look at The Health Foundation (2022) 'What drives Health Inequalities' evidence hub, https://www.health.org.uk/evidence-hub.

For more on poverty look at the Joseph Rowntree Foundation, https://www.jrf.org.uk/.

For more on the Russia-Ukraine conflict, see the United Nations Refugee Agency (UNHCR) portal which is updated weekly at https://data.unhcr.org/en/situations/ukraine.

TEXTBOOKS

Wills, J. (2022). *Foundation for health promotion*. Elsevier, London.
Scriven, A. (2017). *Ewles & Simnett promoting health: A practical guide*. 7th Edition. Elsevier, London.

LISTENING AND WATCHING

Let's Learn Public Health (Australia) with introductory videos to many health promotion concepts at https://www.youtube.com/@LetsLearnPublicHealth.
Resources at the Centers for Disease Control and Prevention (CDC) (US).
Social determinants of health, https://www.youtube.com/watch?v=u_IoBt7Nicw.

How climate affects community health, https://www.youtube.com/watch?v= JywsWktvODc.

Health equity, https://www.youtube.com/watch?v=F8UAanK5WNA.

The Health Foundation (UK) Health inequalities in Scotland: An independent review, https://www.youtube.com/watch?v=GITicmU8g8g, and What makes us healthy? https://www.youtube.com/watch?v=Bnd2Uir_O3g.

'Training in Public Health' (UK) podcast or the John Hopkins Public Health (US) 'Public Health on call' podcast from your podcast provider.

ADDITIONAL REFERENCES

These are the additional references this chapter has used where electronic links have not been provided in the chapter.

Australian Insititute of Health and Welfare. (2023). Health across socio-economic groups. Available at https://www.aihw.gov.au/reports/australias-health/health-across-socioeconomic-groups.

Dahlgren, G., & Whitehead, M. (1991). *Policies and strategies to promote social equity in health.* Institute for Future Studies, Stockholm.

Dahlgren, G., & Whitehead, M. (2021). The Dahlgren-Whitehead model of health determinants: 30 years on and still chasing rainbows. *Public Health, 199,* 20–24. 10.1016/j.puhe.2021.08.009.

Darmody, M., Smyth, E., & Russell, H. (2021). Impacts of the COVID-19 control measures on widening educational inequalities. *Young, 29*(4), 366–380. 10.1177/11033088211027412.

Department of Health (NI). (2022). Health promotion topics. Available at https://www.health-ni.gov.uk/topics/public-health-policy-and-advice/health-promotion.

Department of Health and Social Care. (2021). New TV advert urges the public to stay at home to protect the NHS and save lives. Available at https://www.gov.uk/government/news/new-tv-advert-urges-public-to-stay-at-home-to-protect-the-nhs-and-save-lives.

Ebi, K. L., Capon, A., Berry, P., Broderick, C., de Dear, R., Havenith, G., Honda, Y., Kovats, R. S., Ma, W., Malik, A., Morris, N. B., Nybo, L., Seneviratne, S. I., Vanos, J., & Jay, O. (2021). Hot weather and heat extremes: health risks. *Lancet, 398*(10301), 698–708. 10.1016/s0140-6736(21) 01208-3.

Francis-Devine, B., Harari, D., Keep, M., Bolton, P., Barton, C., & Wilson, W. (2023). Rising cost of living in the UK. House of Commons. Available at https://commonslibrary.parliament.uk/research-briefings/cbp-9428/.

Franklin, B. (1735). On protection of towns from fire, 4 February 1735. Founders Online, National Archives. Available at https://founders.archives.gov/documents/Franklin/01-02-02-0002.

Friebel, R., Molloy, A., Leatherman, S., Dixon, J., Bauhoff, S., & Chalkidou, K. (2018). Achieving high-quality universal health coverage: A perspective from the National Health Service in England. *BMJ Global Health*, *3*(6), e000944. 10.1136/bmjgh-2018-000944.

Gems, G. (2021). *Sport history: The basics*. Routledge, London.

Goldenberg, R. L., McClure, E. M., & Saleem, S. (2018). Improving pregnancy outcomes in low- and middle-income countries. *Reproductive Health*, *15*(1), 88. 10.1186/s12978-018-0524-5.

Government Equalities Office. (2010). Equality Act 2010: Guidance. Available at https://www.gov.uk/guidance/equality-act-2010-guidance.

Government of Canada. (2022). Health promotion. Available at https://www.canada.ca/en/public-health/services/health-promotion.html.

Green, J., Cross, R., Woodall, J., & Tones, K. (2019). *Health promotion: Planning and strategies*. Sage, London.

Heffernan, C. (2019). Fitness and fun that's not just for mum: The Women's League of Health and Beauty in 1930s Ireland. *Women's History Review*, *28*(7), 1017–1038. 10.1080/09612025.2018.1555022.

Hill, L., Ndugga, N., & Artiga, S. (2023). Key data on health and healthcare by race and ethnicity. Available at https://www.kff.org/racial-equity-and-health-policy/report/key-data-on-health-and-health-care-by-race-and-ethnicity/.

Institute of Health Promotion and Health Education. (2021). Position statement. Available at https://ihpe.org.uk/.

International Monetary Fund. (2022). IMF support for fragile and conflict-affected states (FCS). Available at https://www.imf.org/en/Topics/fragile-and-conflict-affected-states.

Jagtap, S., Trollman, H., Trollman, F., Garcia-Garcia, G., Parra-López, C., Duong, L., Martindale, W., Munekata, P. E. S., Lorenzo, J. M., Hdaifeh, A., Hassoun, A., Salonitis, K., & Afy-Shararah, M. (2022). The Russia-Ukraine conflict: Its implications for the global food supply chains. *Foods*, *11*(14). 10.3390/foods11142098.

Jahnel, T., Dassow, H. H., Gerhardus, A., & Schüz, B. (2022). The digital rainbow: Digital determinants of health inequities. *Digital Health*, *8*. 10.1177/20552076221129093.

Joseph Rowntree Foundation. (2023). UK Poverty 2023: The essential guide to understanding poverty in the UK. Available at https://www.jrf.org.uk/report/uk-poverty-2023.

Madsen, W. (2017). Early 20th century conceptualization of health promotion. *Health Promotion International*, *32*(6), 1041–1047. 10.1093/heapro/daw039.

McDaniel, J. T., Nuhu, K., Ruiz, J., & Alorbi, G. (2017). Social determinants of cancer incidence and mortality around the world: An ecological study. *Global Health Promotion*, *26*(1), 41–49. 10.1177/1757975916686913.

National Institute of Clinical Excellence. (2022). *Glossary Health Promotion*. Available at https://www.nice.org.uk/glossary?letter=h.

Nowbar, A. N., Gitto, M., Howard, J. P., Francis, D. P., & Al-Lamee, R. (2019). Mortality from ischemic heart disease. *Circulation: Cardiovascular Quality and Outcomes*, *12*(6), e005375. 10.1161/circoutcomes.118.005375.

OECD. (2019). Health for everyone? Social inequalities in health and health systems. Available at https://www.oecd-ilibrary.org/sites/3c8385d0-en/index.html?itemId=/content/publication/3c8385d0-en.

Office of National Statistics. (2017). Causes of death over 100 years. Available at https://www.ons.gov.uk/peoplepopulationandcommunity/birthsdeathsandmarriages/deaths/articles/causesofdeathover100years/2017-09-18.

Office of National Statistics. (2021). National life tables – Life expectancy in the UK: 2018 to 2020. Available at https://www.ons.gov.uk/peoplepopulationandcommunity/birthsdeathsandmarriages/lifeexpectancies/bulletins/nationallifetablesunitedkingdom/2018to2020.

Office of National Statistics. (2022). Outcomes for disabled people in the UK: 2021. Available at https://www.ons.gov.uk/peoplepopulationandcommunity/healthandsocialcare/disability/articles/outcomesfordisabledpeopleintheuk/2021.

Office of National Statistics. (2023). Coronavirus (COVID-19) latest insights: Infections. Available at https://www.ons.gov.uk/peoplepopulationandcommunity/healthandsocialcare/conditionsanddiseases/articles/coronaviruscovid19latestinsights/infections#long-covid.

Pereira, P., Zhao, W., Symochko, L., Inacio, M., Bogunovic, I., & Barcelo, D. (2022). The Russian-Ukrainian armed conflict will push back the sustainable development goals. *Geography and Sustainability*, *3*(3), 277–287. 10.1016/j.geosus.2022.09.003.

Porter, R. (1999). *Greatest benefit to mankind: Medical history of humanity*. W. W. Norton, London.

Public Health Scotland. (2022). Population health impacts of the rising cost of living in Scotland: A rapid health impact assessment. Available at https://www.publichealthscotland.scot/media/16542/population-health-impacts-of-the-rising-cost-of-living-in-scotland-a-rapid-health-impact-assessment.pdf.

Public Health Wales. (2022). Cost of living crisis in Wales. A public health lens. Available at https://phwwhocc.co.uk/wp-content/uploads/2022/11/PHW-Cost-of-Living-Report-ENG-003.pdf.

Scottish Government. (2018). Scotland's Public Health Priorities. Available at https://www.gov.scot/publications/scotlands-public-health-priorities/pages/1/.

Socialist Health Association. (2022). Peckham experiment. Available at https://www.sochealth.co.uk/national-health-service/public-health-and-wellbeing/peckham-experiment/peckham-experiment-4-in-the-health-centre/.

Swenor, B. K. (2021). Including disability in all health equity efforts: an urgent call to action. *The Lancet Public Health*, *6*(6), e359–e360. 10.1016/S2468-2667(21)00115-8.

Tene, L., Bergroth, T., Eisenberg, A., David, S. S. B., & Chodick, G. (2023). Risk factors, health outcomes, healthcare services utilization, and direct medical costs of patients with long COVID. *International Journal of Infectious Diseases*, *128*, 3–10. 10.1016/j.ijid.2022.12.002.

The Health Foundation. (2022). Evidence hub. Available at https://www.health.org.uk/evidence-hub.

The Health Foundation. (2023). Leave no-one behind. The state of health and health inequalities in Scotland. Available at https://www.health.org.uk/publications/leave-no-one-behind.

Thomson, R. M., Igelström, E., Purba, A. K., Shimonovich, M., Thomson, H., McCartney, G., Reeves, A., Leyland, A., Pearce, A., & Katikireddi, S. V. (2022). How do income changes impact on mental health and wellbeing for working-age adults? A systematic review and meta-analysis. *The Lancet Public Health*, *7*(6), e515–e528. 10.1016/S2468-2667(22)00058-5.

Trust For London. (2022). Life expectancy by London borough. Available at https://www.trustforlondon.org.uk/data/life-expectancy-borough/.

UNHCR. (2023). Ukraine emergency. Available at https://www.unhcr.org/emergencies/ukraine-emergency.

Welshman, J. (1998). Physical culture and sport in schools in England and Wales, 1900–40. *The International Journal of the History of Sport*, *15*(1), 54–75. 10.1080/09523369808714012.

Winchester, N. (2021). Women's health outcomes: Is there a gender gap? Available at https://lordslibrary.parliament.uk/womens-health-outcomes-is-there-a-gender-gap/.

World Economic Forum. (2021). Healthy cities and communities playbook. A white paper by the World Economic forum's platform for shaping the future of consumption. Available at https://www3.weforum.org/docs/WEE_Healthy_Cities_Communities_Playbook_2021.pdf.

World Health Organization. (1948). Constitution of the World Health Organization. Available at http://apps.who.int/gb/bd/.

World Health Organization. (1986). The Ottawa charter for health promotion: First international conference on health promotion, Ottawa, 21 November 1986. Available at https://www.who.int/teams/health-promotion/enhanced-wellbeing/first-global-conference.

World Health Organization. (1997). Jakarta declaration on leading health promotion into the 21st century. Available at https://www.who.int/teams/health-promotion/enhanced-wellbeing/fourth-conference/jakarta-declaration.

World Health Organization. (2010). Adelaide statement on health in all policies. Moving towards a shared governance for health and well-being. Available at https://www.who.int/en/.

World Health Organization. (2016). Shanghai Declaration on promoting health in the 2030 Agenda for Sustainable Development. Available at https://www.who.int/publications/i/item/WHO-NMH-PND-17.5.

World Health Organization. (2020). The top 10 causes of death. Available at https://www.who.int/news-room/fact-sheets/detail/the-top-10-causes-of-death.

World Health Organization. (2023). Climate change. Available at https://www.who.int/health-topics/climate-change.

2

DEVELOPING PERSONAL SKILLS

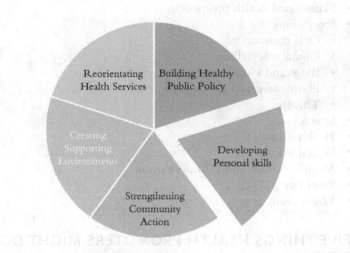

Figure 2.1 Developing personal skills.

- Five things health promoters might do to develop personal skills
- Overview
- The ethics of health promotion
  - Restricting freedom

DOI: 10.4324/9781003462323-3

- Assuming health is easy
- Simplifying complex behaviour
- Unintended consequences
- Health communication
- Communication channels
- New model of communication
- Planning health promotion
- Behaviour change models
- The theory of planned behaviour
- COM–B model
- Why don't people change their behaviour?
- Mass media
- Information technology
- Social Media
- Mobile phones and apps
- Tailoring materials
- Skills–based health promotion
- Storytelling
  - Oral tradition
  - Digital storytelling
  - Blogs and vlogs
  - Photovoice and photodocumentary
  - Theatre
- Literacy
- Health literacy
- Digital literacy
- Misinformation and Disinformation
- Summary
- Wider reading

FIVE THINGS HEALTH PROMOTERS MIGHT DO TO DEVELOP PERSONAL SKILLS

(1) Design and deliver health education in schools or workplaces.
(2) Increase knowledge of health issues through health stands or community events.

(3)   Plan and deliver a health communication campaign through mass media.
(4)   Support people to change their behaviour by offering practical support such as cooking skills or stop smoking support.
(5)   Set up and run community classes for different groups of people to support healthy living such as community walks or gardening groups.

OVERVIEW

People need knowledge and support to change their behaviours. Health promoters can help people to do this in different ways. You might have already been part of the efforts of those already working in health promotion. Perhaps you are wearing a 'smart watch'? That tells you about your steps today? Maybe you have tried the 'Couch to 5k' challenge? https://www.nhs.uk/live-well/exercise/running-and-aerobic-exercises/get-running-with-couch-to-5k/ Given up alcohol for 'Dry January'? https://alcoholchange.org.uk/ Quit smoking on 'Stoptober'? https://thestoptober.co.uk/ Or worn a ribbon for a cancer awareness month? https://www.macmillan.org.uk/cancer-awareness. You might have downloaded an app on your phone, listened to a podcast or watched videos to support a healthy lifestyle change.

Many of the targets in SDG 3 'good health and well-being' require behaviour change support. These include achieving the targets to fight communicable diseases (3.3) reduce mortality from non-communicable diseases and promote mental health (3.4) and prevent substance abuse (3.5). 'Communicable disease' refers to infectious diseases that can be passed from person to person such as HIV and Tuberculosis (TB). 'Non-communicable' diseases are sometimes called 'chronic' diseases or conditions, they are not infectious and include diseases like cancer and diabetes.

Before we explore how health promoters support personal skills development, we need to consider you – the health promoter. The goal of your work is to promote health. This raises questions like: Should we 'make' people change their behaviour? Is this ethical? And what exactly is a 'healthy' lifestyle?

THE ETHICS OF HEALTH PROMOTION

Health promotion action is underpinned by the values or beliefs of a health promoter and their profession. This means that people who work in health promotion have a set of values that inform their actions. If you ask a health promoter why they do their job they might say things like, "I want to make people's health better", "I want to reduce health inequalities" or "I want to improve health in those who are the worst off". Carter et al. (2011) call this a 'normative ideal', meaning health promoters think they can change things in society to make things better. Health promoters may think of one or more of the following:

- That using evidence-based solutions can improve health.
- That some behaviours are 'unhealthy' or 'bad'.
- That if people change their unhealthy behaviours they will be healthier.
- That changes to knowledge, attitudes or beliefs will result in behaviour change.
- That improving the health of one person will affect other people, and thus offer 'collective benefit' to everyone.

These 'normative ideals' inform the way we work. For example, if we deliver information about how and why to breastfeed a baby to an expectant mother, we are assuming that we can encourage a positive attitude towards breastfeeding. We also hope that the mother will believe this is the best option for her and that she will then breastfeed. This will then result in better health outcomes for the baby.

Practitioner skills activity 2a: The value of health.

How much do you value health? Is it something you take for granted? Do you think people value health differently across different age groups? Do you think someone living with a long-term health condition or disability value health differently? Look at the list of 'normative ideals' above. Do you think they would inform your work as a health promoter?

Not everyone values health in the same way as a health promoter. We make assumptions when we design health promotion programmes about what people do (or don't do). Health promoters are in a position of 'power', and we need to make sure we use this power by offering choices or support rather than making someone do something. Remember, health promoters never 'make' anyone do anything. Empowerment is about giving people options. It is not telling someone off or threatening them with terrible consequences if they fail to change. In our enthusiasm, we sometimes forget that not everyone thinks the same way we do.

Health promotion is not always a good thing. Health promotion can restrict people's rights, assume that 'healthy' is easy, simplify complex behaviours, and cause harm. These four issues are discussed below.

RESTRICTING FREEDOM

There is potential for health promotion to restrict or limit the freedoms that people have. For example, the ability of an adult to smoke as many cigarettes as they like is a freedom or right that some people think is 'up to them' or 'their choice'. Saying behaviours are 'unhealthy' or trying to stop them might be taking away something people enjoy, or interfering with people's lives.

ASSUMING HEALTH IS 'EASY'

During the Covid-19 lockdown in the UK in 2020, physical activity was promoted as a good activity to help people stay well. For example, Joe Wicks (The Body Coach) delivered children's physical activity by offering virtual 'PE classes'. You can see the videos at https://www.youtube.com/@TheBodyCoachTV. Whilst many families joined in with the daily classes, widely published campaigns like this often forget that some people might find exercise difficult. They might have no motivation to exercise, have competing priorities, or limited space (Alexander & Shareck, 2021). There are many reasons people find behaviour change hard, and health promoters need to consider ways to support those who find achieving health the hardest.

SIMPLIFYING COMPLEX BEHAVIOUR

Health promotion messages often oversimplify complex behaviours. We cannot reduce obesity simply by telling people to monitor their diet and read food labels. Single interventions that target one behaviour do not impact the things that cause poor health (Laverack, 2017). People may be obese because of a disability, or they live on a low income which restricts food choices. Health promotion action to address obesity should include the other areas of the Ottawa Charter such as campaigning for affordable good quality foods. Simplifying complex behaviours risks blaming or stigmatising people by telling them it is their responsibility to change when they do not have the ability, resources or capacity.

Practitioner skills activity 2b: Why is Evan overweight?

Evan is a 10-year-old boy who is overweight. List at least 10 reasons Evan could be overweight. Look at your list and think about what could stop Evan from taking action to reduce his weight.

UNINTENDED CONSEQUENCES

Health promotion no matter how well-meaning can have unintended consequences. It might cause an injury, or people might stop one behaviour and start a different unhealthy behaviour. For example, someone who quits tobacco smoking might increase their cannabis smoking in response. These risks can sometimes be reduced through good planning and a robust risk assessment.

Empathy is also an important health promotion skill. This is the ability to put yourself in the shoes of another person. This can help you to meet the needs of the people that you are working with. Consider what it might be like to be obese, or live with a mental health condition and think about the assumptions people might make about you. If we cannot empathise with people and their circumstances we risk contributing to the stigma and discrimination people may already experience, and thus worsen health outcomes. An example of discrimination homeless people face in accessing care can be found in Chapter 5 'Reorientating health services'.

HEALTH COMMUNICATION

Health communication is a strategy to deliver health promotion (Corcoran, 2013). An impactful health promoter has good communication skills. This is not just the ability to talk to someone about their health, but also to use the most appropriate 'channels of communication' to deliver information. The design of campaigns, particularly mass media campaigns is also a health communication skill. Health campaigns are the result of what you see on billboards, hear on the radio, read leaflets about or watch on television or social media. Health campaigns are designed to appeal to different audiences and use different formats to communicate health messages. Even when health messages are similar, campaigns choose different ways to appeal to their audiences. See the health promotion in practice example below about mental health promotion.

Health promotion in practice example: Mental health promotion.

Regardless of where we are in the world and who our audiences might be, some health messages are similar. Here are three different examples of mental health videos, all focussed on mental health promotion: If your mates are acting differently, #AskTwice. This part of the 'Time To Change' Mental Health campaign https://www.youtube.com/watch?v=nOkH2jGK4p0. *Billie Eilish On Mental Health & Friendship from the Ad Council (US)* https://www.youtube.com/watch?v=_XFd0RLKQWA. *The World Health Organization video 'I had a black dog, his name was Depression'.* https://www.youtube.com/watch?v=wCd6LPzWscc.

COMMUNICATION CHANNELS

'Channels of communication' are how communication takes place. The people we are trying to reach through these channels are the 'target groups' or 'audience'. Figure 2.2 shows the four channels of communication which are explained below.

- **Intrapersonal** communication channels are one-to-one communication usually through face-to-face conversation.
- **Interpersonal** communication is conversations between peers, or in a small group.
- **Organisation** communication channels use key leaders or influencers such as faith leaders, or employers, to send messages.
- **Mass media** communication includes information technology and social media. This is covered later in the chapter.

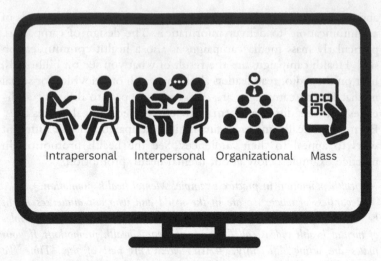

Figure 2.2 Channels of communication.

In health promotion, multiple channels of communication can be used to deliver health promotion. For example, in a school, mass media resources could be used with young people when teaching about alcohol harm, but a mental health support group might meet face-to-face and use social media.

Health promoters choose the right channels of communication for their work. We ask questions like, what information do we need to deliver? Which format will work best? And where will my target group be most likely to engage with my messages or campaign? For example, this YouTube video delivers brief sexual health information through a quiz, https://www.youtube.com/watch?v=2Y4g88KC6V4 but this NHS website is more like an online magazine https://www.healthforteens.co.uk/sexual-health/. Choosing the right channel increases the chances that your target group will see your message and engage with the content.

Practitioner skills activity 2c: Channels of communication.

You want to improve oral health in children in a primary school aged 5–11 years. You have chosen to deliver a toothbrushing campaign. This campaign trains teachers to run oral health education classes for children as well as supervised teeth brushing in the classroom every day. Parents will receive health education on how to support their children's oral health at home. What channels of communication would you use for teachers, children and parents? The channels of communication will likely be different for different groups.

A NEW MODEL OF COMMUNICATION

In health promotion, we assume that when we give information to people they will do something with the information. For example, the target group will read the leaflet, watch the health campaign video and then act on that information. In reality, many people don't. Look at Figure 2.3 and read the things that people say in a message about doing 30 minutes of physical activity five times a week. It shows that people are not listening, don't understand or are confused about the message. It is difficult to send a message that will be understood or relevant to everyone.

These are the challenges that health promoters face:

- Challenge 1: Reaching people with a message they understand and listen to. Messages can also be misunderstood, ignored, irrelevant, unachievable or boring.
- Challenge 2: Encouraging people to act on the message. It may mean people have to give up things they like or do something they find hard.

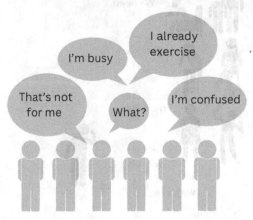

Figure 2.3 Different responses to health promotion messages.

- Challenge 3: That the message is culturally relevant. The creators of messages are often health promoters or groups of people who are different to the target group they are trying to reach.

Most health messages come from the 'top-down'. This is when a health promoter (at the top) designs a message and delivers it to a target group (at the bottom). This suggests health promoters know best, when they may not. A 'bottom-up' approach to health communication places the target group at the top. They become the ones who create the messages, rather than the health promoter. Figure 2.4 shows this 'user-led' approach.

Figure 2.4 suggests that the target group chooses the health priorities, the communication channels and designs (or gives ideas for the design) of messages. The health promoter is the listener, advocator or facilitator who crafts these ideas into actions. Most people are quite able to identify their health needs and say what needs to be different. Designing messages based on what people say helps to reflect the way people live. If we spent more time working with target groups to explore their ideas then our messages would be more meaningful.

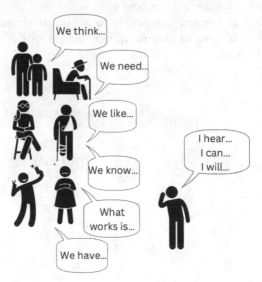

Figure 2.4 User-led model of health communication.

PLANNING HEALTH PROMOTION

To design a health promotion intervention or programme we need to know:

- What is the health issue we intend to address?
- What do we aim to do with the health issue (reduce, increase, prevent)?
- What best practice solution(s) can we use?

For example, if we wanted to focus on tobacco smoking, we need information like who smokes, why they smoke and how much they smoke. We need to decide what we aim to do. Is it to stop people from starting smoking or encourage people who smoke to quit? We also want to know what solutions could be used to achieve our aim.

Health promoters usually use a planning model to help them design a campaign. These are the main steps in a planning model.

- **Rationale:** This section uses data and evidence to say why the health issue needs to be addressed.
- **Target group:** This is the audience that your campaign is aimed at.
- **Aim:** This is what your campaign intends to do.
- **Methods, design, settings, stakeholders:** This is a plan of what you will do, who is involved and how you will do it.
- **Resources, time frame and budget:** This is what resources you need to deliver your campaign, how much they will cost and how long it will take to do your campaign.
- **Evaluation:** This measures the value of the campaign and whether it worked.

You can have a look at some of the health promotion planning models in the wider reading list at the end of the chapter. For more on evaluation, see Chapter 6 'Reorientating health services'.

Practitioner skills activity 2d: Using evidence to decide on a target group.
Smoking rates in UK adults are around 13 to 15% (around 6 million adults) (Office for Health Improvement and Disparities, 2022). More men than women smoke and white ethnicities smoke more than other ethnic

groups. 25–34-year-olds have the highest rate of current smoking, and those with no qualifications are more likely to smoke. 16–24 years are more likely to vape or use e-cigarettes (Office of National Statistics, 2021). Using the information above, who would you target group for a campaign, and why?

BEHAVIOUR CHANGE MODELS

When we plan health promotion we try to predict what we think stops people from doing healthy behaviours or what puts people at higher risk of getting ill or dying. This is difficult, so health promoters use health behaviour change theories or models to help. These theories offer a way of understanding what influences people's behaviours. These 'influencers' are then targeted in interventions to try and encourage behaviour change.

The most commonly used behaviour change theories and models come from the field of health psychology. The models include the Health Belief Model (Becker, 1974), the Transtheoretical model (or Stages of Change model) (Prochaska & Diclemente, 1983), the Theory of Planned Behaviour (Ajzen, 1991), Social Learning Theory (Bandura, 1988) and the Com-B model (Michie et al., 2014). As this book is an introduction to health promotion and these models are quite complex, I have chosen two models to show you how behaviour change models work. There is a 'Health Psychology: The Basics' book in the same series as this book which covers some of these models in much more detail. There are also wider reading resources for health promotion theories at the end of the chapter.

THE THEORY OF PLANNED BEHAVIOUR

The theory of planned behaviour (TPB) (Ajzen, 1991) states that attitude, subjective norm and perceived behavioural control influence behavioural intention and that this influences behaviour. The TPB can be seen in Figure 2.5.

- Attitude is someone's positive or negative feelings towards something.
- Subjective norm is the influence of significant others like friends and family.

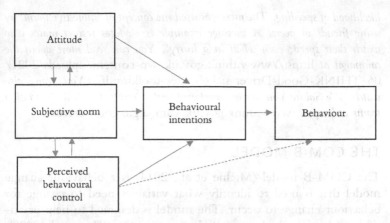

Figure 2.5 The Theory of Planned Behaviour, adapted from Ajzen (1991).

- Perceived behaviour control is how much control people feel they have over doing a behaviour.
- Behavioural intention is the intention that someone has to do the behaviour.

The model suggests that the more positive the attitude, the more supportive the subjective norm, the higher the perceived ability to do the behaviour, and the more likely the intention to do the behaviour, the more likely it is a person will do the behaviour. Take the example of wearing a seatbelt in a car. The more that you believe a seatbelt is a good thing and that it will protect you (attitude), the more others wear a seatbelt or tell you to wear a seatbelt (subjective norm) the more you find wearing a seatbelt easy to do (perceived behavioural control), the more likely you will intend to wear one (behaviour intention), and consequently wear one (behaviour). The example of the THINK! 'good driver campaign' below also shows how this model works.

Health promotion in practice example: 'THINK! Good driver campaign (UK).

The THINK! Good driver campaign focussed on 17 to 24-year-old male drivers. These drivers are more likely to be killed or seriously injured than drivers 25 years or over. In THINK research they found higher acceptability of mobile phone use without a handsfree device while driving, and a higher likelihood of speeding. The messages used the concept of 'subjective norm' by using friends or peers. A message example is: 'Mates respect mates who watch their speed, even when in a hurry'. You can read more about the campaign at https://www.think.gov.uk/wp-content/uploads/2021/06/THINK-Good-Driver-stakeholder-toolkit.pdf. *You can also watch 'We Salute You' a film developed with County Football Association teams at* https://www.think.gov.uk/campaign/good-driver/.

THE COM-B MODEL

The COM-B model (Michie et al., 2014) is a behaviour change model that is used to identify what variables need to change for behaviour change to occur. The model is designed to help practitioners identify which areas of change to target (West et al., 2020). This model has three factors that are important for a behaviour change to take place. These are illustrated in Figure 2.6.

Figure 2.6 shows the three factors important to behaviour change in the COM-B model, and the two strands that make up each of the three factors. The three factors are capability, opportunity and motivation.

- **Capability** is the ability to 'do' the behaviour.
- **Opportunity** is the external chance to 'do' the behaviour.
- **Motivation** is the internal desire to 'do' the behaviour.

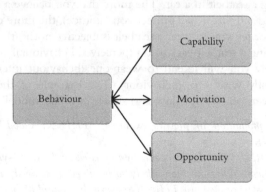

Figure 2.6 The COM-B model, adapted from Michie et al. (2014).

This is an example of how the model might work for going to the gym to exercise regularly. To go to a gym to exercise three times a week a person would need to be able to use the equipment in a gym (capability), to have the time, money and access to facilities to go to a gym (opportunity), and to want to go to the gym or go regularly and form the habit of going (motivation). See also the health promotion example below.

Health promotion in practice example: COM-B and Covid-19 preventive behaviours.

During Covid-19 the authors of the COM-B argue that many behaviours could be targeted using their model. For example, for wearing and using a face mask correctly people may need to:

- *Understand what mask to use, when to use it, and how to use it = Capability.*
- *Have masks available or the facilities to make them = Opportunity.*
- *Ensure that wearing a mask still means people comply with other measures like social distancing, and that people wear marks correctly and do not touch or remove them to talk to someone = Motivation.*

For more examples of applying the principles of behaviour change to reduce Covid-19 see https://www.nature.com/articles/s41562-020-0887-9.

The model also breaks down each of the three factors (capability, opportunity and motivation) into two strands.

- **Capability** is split into **physical capability** and **psychological capability**. Physical capability is the ability of that person to have the physical skills to do a behaviour, for example having good balance or coordination. Psychological capability is a person's mental functioning ability such as being able to understand an instruction.
- **Opportunity** is split into **physical opportunity** and **social opportunity**. Physical opportunities are factors such as time or money. Social opportunity involves other people such as social influences or group norms.
- **Motivation** is split into **reflective motivation** and **autonomic motivation**. Reflective motivation is conscious thought processes such as being able to plan. Autonomic motivation is the habits or instincts of things we do.

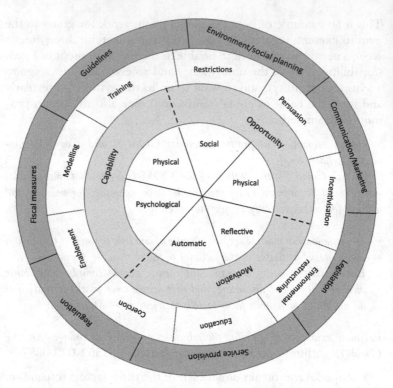

Figure 2.7 The Behaviour Change Wheel, adapted from Michie et al. (2014).

Splitting the components of capability, opportunity and motivation allows practitioners to match interventions to different aspects of behaviour. These three components work alongside a behaviour change wheel. The behaviour change wheel has nine intervention functions and seven policy categories. There are training and resources available for how to use the behaviour change wheel (see below). Figure 2.7 shows the behaviour change wheel.

The behaviour change wheel in Figure 2.7 shows 'nine intervention functions' which are ways of targeting Capability, Opportunity and Motivation to support behaviour change. These are the middle layers of the wheel and include: education, persuasion, incentivisation, coercion, training, enablement, modelling, environmental restricting and restrictions. The behaviour change wheel also identifies seven policy categories that support the delivery of the intervention functions. These are: environmental/social planning, communication/ marketing, legislation, service provision, regulation, fiscal measures and guidelines.

The process of using the behaviour change wheel is quite complex. However, here are two examples to give you an idea of how the behaviour change wheel works in cancer screening services:

Example 1: A health professional identifies that women are not attending breast cancer screening as they have to travel long distances to reach screening services (physical opportunity). To increase the uptake of screening services mobile screening centres placed closer to where people live could be used (from the seven policy categories this would be environmental/social planning).

Example 2: A health professional wants to increase uptake of bowel cancer screening, and identifies that people are not returning the home test kits. In the UK these tests are called the 'faecal immunochemical test' (FIT). Exploration of why the kits are not being returned finds that people do not understand the instructions (psychological capability). To increase the number of people returning test kits, a video could be used to show people what to do (from the nine intervention functions this is modelling) like this NHS video on doing the FIT test https://www.youtube.com/watch?v=Hb7euOEXEsc.

To learn more about the training and resource book for the behaviour change wheel see http://www.behaviourchangewheel.com/.

WHY DON'T PEOPLE CHANGE THEIR BEHAVIOUR?

Even when we carefully plan health promotion, use evidence, and use health promotion theory our efforts do not always work. This can be very frustrating for the health promoter, but there are many reasons people do not change. A person might like doing an 'unhealthy' behaviour, for example drinking alcohol every day. They may lack the motivation to change behaviours. People may not know when a good time to change is, or what needs to change. It also might be difficult to keep a behaviour going all the time.

Practitioner skills activity 2e: Differences in behaviour.
Have a look at the Covid-19 map from the Institute of Health Metrics and Evaluation of those who wore masks when going out in 2021 at https://www.healthdata.org/acting-data/covid-19-maps-mask-use. Why do you think there are such variations in countries between those who wore marks and those who did not? What reasons can you see why people did not want to wear a mask even if it was recommended?

Behaviour is closely connected to our social circumstances and living conditions. Inequalities in these areas like living in unsafe communities or not being able to work can mean behaviour change is a challenge. Health promoters should focus on those who need the most support first so we don't risk leaving people behind. See the example below of the 'baby box' scheme which aims to support new babies to get an equal start in life.

Health promotion in practice example: Baby box initiatives.
Baby box initiatives are designed to give all babies an equal start in life. A baby box is a maternity package that contains products for a new baby, as well as maternity items. The original Babybox scheme started in Finland. You can see what is in the most recent maternity box and read more at https://www.kela.fi/maternitypackage. Although items vary, the box itself is intended as a baby bed, and products include things like a blanket, towel, baby clothes, baby care items and hygiene products. There are different versions of the baby box scheme in other countries, for example, Babybox Canada at https://babyboxcanada.org/ and Scotland's Babybox at https://www.mygov.scot/baby-box.

MASS MEDIA

Mass media is widely used in health promotion. It is any type of media including printed, electronic, audio or visual. It is usually formed of one or two messages aimed at the general public, often without ever seeing the audience. It is not a magic bullet that instantly changes behaviour, although this idea still exists in the heads of some who are looking for an easy option to promote health. Mass media has strengths and weaknesses.

- Mass media can increase knowledge, raise awareness, convey simple messages, get people talking about health and support people who are ready to change.

- Mass media is not so good at giving complicated information or instructions, changing strongly held beliefs or supporting behaviour change without other resources.

Mass media today is mainly used in health promotion to increase knowledge or raise awareness of a health issue or service. For example, the NHS 111 'Help Us Help You' campaign is designed to encourage the general public to use the NHS 111 online service when they think they need medical help. See the campaign toolkit and resources at https://campaignresources.phe.gov.uk/resources/campaigns/119--nhs-111-online-2022.

Health promotion in practice example: Stroke and FAST.

Research suggests that stroke outcomes are better when medical help is obtained quickly. Act FAST is a stroke campaign in the UK which aims to encourage people to act FAST when they see the symptoms of a stroke. It was relaunched in 2021 after data showed that hospital admissions for stroke reduced during the Covid-19 pandemic (Public Health England, 2021). F.A.S.T. stands for face, arms, speech and time.

- *Face: Has their face fallen or drooped?*
- *Arm: Can they raise both their arms?*
- *Speech: Is their speech slurred?*
- *Time: Time to call 999 if they see any of these signs.*

The Stroke Association also has resources for FAST at https://www.stroke.org.uk/what-is-stroke/what-are-the-symptoms-of-stroke.

In 2019, World Stroke Day created 'FAST Heros', a global school-based campaign to raise awareness of stroke in schools (World Stroke Organization, 2023). See more at https://www.world-stroke.org/world-stroke-day-campaign/why-stroke-matters/stroke-treatment/signs-of-stroke-fast. *Globally, other countries also use FAST to increase knowledge of stroke and the importance of seeking urgent medical care, for example, New Zealand* https://www.stroke.org.nz/fast *and America (USA)* https://www.stroke.org/en/help-and-support/resource-library/fast-materials

Mass media can convey simple messages and get people talking about health. For example, the podcast (an audio programme in a digital format), 'You, me and the Big C: Putting the Can in Cancer' is a BBC podcast about cancer run by people living with cancer.

You can listen to the podcasts at https://www.bbc.co.uk/ programmes/p0608649/episodes/downloads. More podcast examples can be found in the 'tailoring materials' section later in this chapter. Mass media can also motivate people to change when people feel supported or ready to act. Think of the examples at the start of this chapter like 'Couch to 5k' which encourages people to move from the couch to running 5 kilometres.

Mass media is not very good at telling people complicated information or instructions. Think about the last time you tried to remember what items you needed in the supermarket! It cannot change strongly held beliefs, for example about the transmission of disease. It cannot change behaviour if there are no other 'enabling' factors to support change. For example, it would be difficult to take up handwashing for infection control in the absence of soap and water.

Health promotion in practice example: Livelighter® Australia.

Livelighter® is a mass media campaign for obesity prevention in Western Australia. The website focuses on healthy eating, healthy cooking and shopping smart. The campaign website includes recipes, calculators, meal plans, workout guides and other resources. There are several evaluations of the campaign which has been running since 2012. One of the most recent evaluations suggests the campaign is good value for money as part of broader evidence-based obesity prevention strategies (Ananthapavan et al., 2022). You can read more about the campaign at https://livelighter.com.au/.

Mass media, like health promotion, is more successful when it has a supportive environment. For example, SDG target 12.5 is focused on reducing waste through reduction, recycling and reuse. A campaign to try and achieve this would be more successful if it looked at both the individual and the settings in which they live. Messages that focus on climate change behaviours such as using less plastic are stronger when supported by policies that reduce plastic use. Bans on plastic straws or cutlery, or stores charging a plastic bag fee support behaviour change. See the health promotion in practice example below for an example of using mass media to reduce child exploitation.

Health promotion in practice example: Operation Makesafe (England).

Operation Makesafe was designed by the Metropolitan Police with London Boroughs to raise awareness of child exploitation in the business community such as hotels, licensed premises like pubs and nightclubs, taxi companies and shops.

Resources are aimed at increasing community and organisation awareness of child exploitation. You can watch the video at this link https://www.youtube.com/watch?v=7Izq9SosOGE *and see the resources at* https://www.met.police.uk/police-forces/metropolitan-police/areas/about-us/about-the-met/campaigns/operation-makesafe/.

INFORMATION TECHNOLOGY

Information technology (IT) includes the internet, social media platforms and mobile phones. Figure 2.8 shows you some of the different ways that IT is used in health promotion. This includes social media, videos, podcasts, blogs, the internet and providing support via chats or email.

IT also has the benefit of being interactive for the user. For example, the website 'Love Food Hate Waste', allows the user to search for recipes by typing in the food they have left over to help them reduce food waste. See more at https://www.lovefoodhatewaste.com/. Many organisations offer online communities, for example, 'The Stroke Association' has online forums through 'my stroke guide' as well as an online activities hub that supports people through exercises, drop-ins, quizzes and games. You can see more at https://www.stroke.org.uk/finding-support/my-stroke-guide.

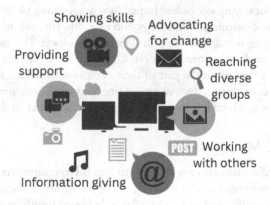

Showing skills

Advocating for change

Providing support

Reaching diverse groups

Working with others

Information giving

Figure 2.8 Information Technology in health promotion.

IT can support skill development by showing skills either live or pre-recorded. See the practitioner skills activity below on learning cardiopulmonary resuscitation (CPR).

Practitioner skills activity 2f: Learn CPR to music.

CPR (cardiopulmonary resuscitation) is when you give chest compressions to someone in cardiac arrest to keep them alive until help like the emergency services arrive. You can learn this lifesaving skill on the internet. The British Heart Foundation provides resources to help you learn CPR in 15 minutes at https://www.bhf.org.uk/how-you-can-help/how-to-save-a-life/how-to-do-cpr *There are videos and other resources as well as a link to songs where you can practice the CPR rhythm (100–120 beats per minute).*

For health promoters, the internet provides resources to support your practice. For example, 'Boost' is a mobile resource for community workers and peer educators in South and East Africa. It provides teaching resources and activities for HIV, sexual health and Covid-19. It is free to download and can be used offline. See https://boost.avert.org/. The British Heart Foundation provides resources to anyone working with those with, or at risk of, heart disease at https://www.bhf.org.uk/for-professionals/healthcare-professionals.

There are challenges to using IT. Cybercrime and cyberbullying for example are only possible because of our digital world, and finding ways to reduce these is a challenge. Some people may be more vulnerable than others to cybercrime. For example, Age UK has resources for older people about staying safe online https://www.ageuk.org.uk/information-advice/work-learning/technology-internet/internet-security/.

Cyberbullying is bullying through digital technology. The rise of social media has made this more common. UNICEF has a resource for young people on cyberbullying as part of their campaign to reduce it. You can read more at https://www.unicef.org/end-violence/how-to-stop-cyberbullying. There is a section on 'digital literacy' later in this chapter.

SOCIAL MEDIA

Social media platforms are a space to reach large numbers of people and offer potential health promotion opportunities. Social media is most commonly used to increase knowledge of health issues or offer support. Ghahramani et al. (2022) suggest that social media can be used to increase reach, exposure, impact and engagement in health promotion campaigns, and thus should be a consideration in mass media campaigns.

Although there are many different types of social media, platforms that provide support for videos or provide spaces for discussions are the most popular. There are several roles for health promoters in using social media. Stellefson et al. (2020) outline several ways including:

- Engaging with stakeholders and advocates. This might be to get support for health campaigns or policies by interacting with others.
- Being aware of how your target audiences use social media. This helps to target messages appropriately.
- Delivering social media messages effectively. This includes adopting best practice guidelines for using social media.
- Evaluating the health messages that circulate on social media. This means monitoring and evaluating social media messages for reach, impact or effectiveness.

Practitioner skills activity 2g: Using social media.

If you use social media look at the different support groups that are available for the health issues that you are interested in. If you don't have any social media accounts look at places like 'YouTube' which do not require an account. You could also search for health podcasts or look at large organisations on Facebook without creating a social media account. For example The British Red Cross https://www.facebook.com/BritishRedCross/ or Macmillan Cancer Support https://en-gb.facebook.com/macmillancancer/.

MOBILE PHONES AND APPS

Mobile phones can be used for basic information giving in the form of text messages such as appointments, contraception or medication reminders or giving test results. For example, mobile phones can be used to support 'Directly observed treatment, short-course' (DOTS) to observe or remind people living with Tuberculosis (TB) to take their daily medication. It can also help to reduce 'no-show' healthcare appointments.

Practitioner skills activity 2h: Quality of health apps.

There is a large variation in the quality of health apps. In the UK, ORCHA is an organisation that reviews and approves apps for use in the NHS. They have an App Finder which means you can access reviews of different apps across many different health conditions. Northwest London NHS have an App Finder and a video about the ORCHA review process. Use this link and search for a health condition like diabetes or depression to see what apps are recommended at https://nwlhealthapps.orcha.co.uk/.

Mobile phones can also provide alerts or notifications, for example, weather risks or emergency alerts. There are also numerous apps available for download to calculate alcohol units, count calories, check sexual health symptoms, count steps, track physical activity, check balance and monitor mood. They can also deliver programmes of support over time. For example, the NHS-recommended sleep app 'Sleepio' is a six-week sleep improvement programme. See more at https://www.sleepio.com/.

Health promotion in practice example: Women's health apps.

'Balance' is a menopause app. It allows users to track symptoms, measure mood, read expert advice, share stories in a community of users, and download a health report. Read more at https://www.balance-menopause.com/balance-app/

'MomConnect' is an M-Health intervention in South Africa to promote better maternal health in pregnancy through mobile phones. It registers pregnancies, can send targeted health promotion messages and provides support. Read more at https://www.health.gov.za/momconnect/

TAILORING MATERIALS

Tailoring information is when health information is adapted to ensure it meets the needs of different groups of people. This can make it more culturally relevant or target messages at specific 'at risk' populations. IT has the potential to tailor information to groups of people without the need for another set of campaign messages. Terrance Higgins Trust (THT) for example, has information for being tested for HIV, being diagnosed with HIV, and living well with HIV. People seeking information do not all have the same HIV status or information needs. Read more at https://www.tht.org.uk/hiv-and-sexual-health. Macmillan cancer support also provides a list of resources for people living with the many different types of cancers https://www. macmillan.org.uk/cancer-information-and-support/cancer-types.

Other websites can tailor information to specific people using interactive activities. For example, Diabetes UK allows you to calculate your risk of Type 2 diabetes through a series of questions. You can do this at https://riskscore.diabetes.org.uk/start, it then offers advice based on the information you give. The NHS has a similar resource to calculate your heart age at https://www.nhs.uk/health-assessment-tools/calculate-your-heart-age. Another example is 'mind plans' in practitioner skills activity 2i.

Other forms of media like podcasts can create content to reach specific populations, for example 'the disability and' podcasts to support those living with a disability, 'Life after Prison' for those who have left prison or 'Pumping Marvellous' to support people with living with heart failure. See the links at the end of the chapter.

Practitioner skills activity 2i: Mind plans (England).

The Better Health – Every Mind Matters NHS campaign encourages adults to complete a 'mind plan', which gives a personalised mental health action plan with practical tips for dealing with stress, mood, sleep etc. Complete the NHS Mind-Plan at https://www.nhs.uk/every-mind-matters/mental-wellbeing-tips/your-mind-plan-quiz/.

SKILLS-BASED HEALTH PROMOTION

Teaching skills to help support people to change their behaviour is an important part of health promotion. This means people are more empowered to make changes for themselves. For example, if you had no cooking skills and you were reading instructions about what to do with an onion, what is the difference between chopped, diced, minced and sliced? What does soften, sauté, fry or sweat mean? By demonstrating cooking skills face to face, or through videos, it can be much easier to support people to develop knowledge and confidence.

'We are undefeatable' is a website that encourages physical activity in those living with a health condition and includes workout videos and resources https://weareundefeatable.co.uk/. Other websites focus on skill-building through toolkits. For example, the British Red Cross has kindness packs to try and build confidence and resilience, improve general well-being and reduce loneliness.

View resources at https://www.redcross.org.uk/get-help/get-help-with-loneliness/wellbeing-support.

Teaching people in small groups in settings such as schools or working in communities on community projects can support people to live well. A project that builds skills in peers and family members is shown in the Naloxone example below. Community projects are covered in more detail in Chapter 3 'Strengthening community action'.

Health promotion in practice example: Training drug users to use Naloxone (Scotland).

Accidental overdose is a common cause of death among users of heroin or other opioids. Naloxone is an essential medicine for the treatment of opioid overdose and it can reverse the effects of an overdose. The purpose of Naloxone is to provide time for emergency services to arrive and for further treatment to be given. The concept of 'take home' Naloxone means the provision of an emergency supply of Naloxone to be given to peers, family members or other non-medical people who may be likely to witness an opioid overdose. They are trained in giving the drug in an emergency. Scotland was one of the first countries to introduce a national Naloxone programme which includes peer training, increasing access to Naloxone and campaign awareness materials (Scottish Government, 2022). Read more at https://www.stopthedeaths.com/.

STORYTELLING

Storytelling is a way of communicating which can help us make sense of our world (Lipsey et al., 2020). Storytelling in health uses stories that may involve real or fictitious people and situations to talk about health. This might be through a play, drama or orally sharing a story. This has many potential benefits for health education as diverse topics can be included and stories can be designed to appeal to different population groups. Storytelling has also been used as a psychological intervention such as sharing stories of trauma, and to advocate for change. For example, Mwaba et al. (2021) use storytelling as a form of activism to prevent violence against women in Turkey. There are many examples of the way storytelling is used in health promotion research and practice. Figure 2.9 illustrates some of the ways that stories can be told about health. It shows oral tradition, digital storytelling, blogs or vlogs, photovoice and photodocumentary and theatre, all of which are discussed more below.

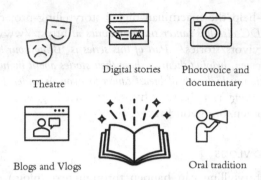

Figure 2.9 Examples of ways stories can be told about health.

ORAL TRADITION

Storytelling using the oral tradition may not just be stories as we think of them in books, but also singing, chanting, poems and rhymes. The role of a storyteller is usually to educate and entertain an audience so the stories may not be true although they may have a moral or educational purpose. Stories can tell us about the real world and how people cope, live and overcome challenges. For example, TedX has a resource with 'personal stories from Conflict Zones' https://www.ted.com/playlists/481/personal_stories_from_conflict and a talk on 'why we tell stories at https://www.ted.com/playlists/756/why_do_we_tell_stories.

DIGITAL STORYTELLING

People tell short stories to others through digital visual means. They tell the story from the person's point of view which can 'elevate voices' that are not usually heard (Lohr et al., 2022). Digital storytelling has been used in many different contexts. For example, in Uganda, it has been used to promote child health. See https://www.healthychilduganda.org/digital-stories/. See the health promotion in practice example for how it has been used for cancer.

Health promotion in practice example: Digital storytelling for cancer.

In the UK, Macmillan has a digital storytelling project at https://www.macmillan.org.uk/cancer-information-and-support/get-help/

emotional-help/the-macmillan-digital-storytelling-project. *In the US, the CDC also has cancer survivor stories at* https://www.cdc.gov/cancer/survivors/stories/. *Part of this series is 'Bring your brave' aimed at young women, helping them to share their stories about living with breast cancer or being at high risk of breast cancer for women under 45 years. See more about Bring Your Brave at* https://www.cdc.gov/cancer/breast/young_women/bringyourbrave/.

BLOGS AND VLOGS

Personal storytelling can happen through text (blogs) and videos (vlogs). These are published on websites or spaces such as 'YouTube'. It is a way of sharing personal health stories with others such as living with a long-term illness such as diabetes or being pregnant for the first time. An example is the 'Health stories project'. This is a voluntary organisation publishing stories and photographs from people who are living with long-term or chronic illnesses. You can read more at https://healthstoriesproject.com/.

PHOTOVOICE AND PHOTODOCUMENTARY

Photodocumentary is when a storyteller tries to tell something using photographs, often with accompanying text. One of the pioneers of photodocumentary is Dorothea Lange who was hired to document the effects of the Depression in America. Her 1936 'Migrant Mother' (California) photograph tells of the hardships of impoverished migrant farmers. You can see this at https://www.moma.org/learn/moma_learning/dorothea-lange-migrant-mother-nipomo-california-1936/.

Photovoice also uses photographs to tell a story but aims to put the camera in the hands of people to show their experiences. This is based on techniques by Wang et al. (1998) and is participatory in nature. It asks participants to tell stories about their lives, usually to advocate for change. It is most often used as a research method for change, for example, the photovoice 'Villaverde' exploring food environments in Madrid (Díaz et al., 2021). You can see more on this at https://www.youtube.com/watch?v=VIiFggKzVas and the 'Health Heart Hoods' website at https://www.hhhproject.es/.

THEATRE

Theatre, plays or drama can tell or show stories about health. Theatre can give us different perspectives on health as we watch or listen to a story unfold and follow characters as they make decisions throughout the play. There are many examples of the ways drama or theatre is used in health education. An example from India is the use of street plays to promote eye health awareness (Pehere & Yadavalli, 2021) and in Australia theatre has been used for 'bystander interventions' to change attitudes to gender-based violence (Crisp & Taket, 2022). The theatre company 'Odd Arts' in Manchester (UK) delivers theatre to support mental health for those at greatest risk of inequalities and discrimination including in criminal justice systems. See more at https://oddarts.co.uk. See the health promotion in practice example below for theatre in health education for young people.

Health promotion in practice example: Theatre in education for young people.

In New Zealand, the Theatre in Education Trust (THETA) provides health education programmes for young people through theatre. 'Sexwise' uses songs, humour, drama and discussion for rangatahi/youth across New Zealand in years 9–13 in secondary schools. It follows four typical teenagers and their relationships through play and workshops. You can see more including videos at https://sexwise.nz/ *and other THETA programmes at* https://thetanewzealand.github.io/. *In Birmingham (England) the theatre company 'Loudmouth' delivers a wide variety of educational programmes through theatre around bullying, safeguarding and young people's health. See more at* https://www.loudmouth.co.uk/.

LITERACY

Literacy is the skills to read, write, speak and listen effectively and to use this to make sense of what is going on around us (National Literacy Trust, 2023). Not having these skills is associated with inequalities such as lack of access to education and employment. It also puts people at higher risk of poorer health outcomes. In England, data shows that those who are older, and those out of work are more likely to have low literacy or numeracy skills (Learning and Work Institute, 2022). Improving literacy and numeracy skills is important in helping to reduce inequalities in the social determinants of health. See the health promotion in practice example below about prisoners and prison radio.

Health promotion in practice example: Literacy and National Prison Radio.

On average, the literacy levels of prisoners are lower than that of the general population. Improving the literacy of those in prisons can support people to learn skills and get work when they are released (UK Government, 2022). 'National Prison Radio' produces programmes that target key factors linked to reducing people's likelihood of reoffending. These include exercise programmes, motivational talk shows and support for life after prison. One programme 'Books Unlocked' aims to make books more accessible to prisoners and young offenders across England and Wales. To read more about National Prison Radio see https://prison.radio/national-prison-radio/, *to read more about Books Unlocked see* https://literacytrust.org.uk/programmes/books-unlocked/. *You can also read about National Prison Radio in many different countries including Australia, the Republic of Ireland, Trinidad and Tobago, Sweden, India and Norway at* https://prison.radio/prison-radio-international/.

HEALTH LITERACY

The ability of people to understand and use health information is 'health literacy'. Improving health literacy means people can understand health information that is important to them, as well as support them to manage their health. Health literacy is not simply reading and writing, but about what literacy enables us to do. Freebody & Luke (1990) argue that literacy skills like reading and writing are social activities or social practices, and therefore not being able to do them means not being able to participate in those activities where reading and writing are important. Nutbeam (2000) develops this further by suggesting three types of literacy categories that can be applied to health: functional, interactive and critical. These are illustrated in Figure 2.10 with examples.

As illustrated in Figure 2.10, functional health literacy is the basic literacy skill needed to get health information. Interactive health literacy is more advanced and is the skill to extract information and take meaning from this. It is about being able to take information

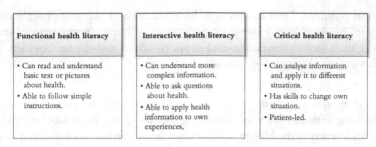

Functional health literacy	Interactive health literacy	Critical health literacy
• Can read and understand basic text or pictures about health. • Able to follow simple instructions.	• Can understand more complex information. • Able to ask questions about health. • Able to apply health information to own experiences.	• Can analyse information and apply it to different situations. • Has skills to change own situation. • Patient-led.

Figure 2.10 Three strands of health literacy.

and apply it to different situations, as well as engaging with health professionals such as asking questions. Critical health literacy is the ability to analyse and apply health information across different life events and experiences. More advanced cognitive skills are needed for this.

Health literacy is a determinant of health and there are inequalities in who is health literate (Nutbeam & Lloyd, 2021). People with lower levels of literacy and health literacy may have more difficulties accessing health information, understanding and applying health information, and using available information to prevent ill health and manage health conditions. To reduce inequalities we need to increase health literacy, and this means improving the quality of health communication and the people it reaches, as well as developing individuals' transferable skills. Transferable skills are life skills such as problem solving and analysing information. These skills are needed to locate and use health information. For example, understanding medication doses, times and number of tablets as well as when to take it requires numeracy skills, such as telling the time or calculating how much to take. Health literacy skills are also important in being able to identify misinformation or disinformation. This is discussed below.

The World Health Organization (2022) has a resource on developing health literacy skills for non-communicable diseases with global case studies at https://www.who.int/publications/i/item/9789240055391. 'Change' is a human rights charity led by disabled people. Their resource highlights how and why 'Easy Read' materials are important for inclusion and equity https://www.changepeople.org/our-work/easy-read-portfolio. Their resources include Macmillan Cancer Support 'Easy read' booklets like 'Having an ultrasound' at https://www.macmillan.org.uk/cancer-information-and-support/stories-and-media/booklets/having-an-ultrasound-easy-read.

Practitioner skills activity 2j: Teach back method.

A method that health promoters use to ensure that the person they are working with has understood health information is the 'teach back' method. This is a way of checking to see if someone has understood, and that they can show you or 'teach back' the information. For example, a health practitioner might say "I have given you a lot of information today. Can you tell me what three things you need to do next …" or, "To make sure I have explained everything clearly, can you tell me what you are going to do with this medicine each day".

You are working with Mary. She is living with diabetes, and you want to explain to her why it is important that she measures her blood pressure frequently. You want to suggest ways she can reduce her blood pressure through the foods she eats. Give some examples of what you could say to Mary, using the 'teach back' method. To read more on managing blood pressure with diabetes see https://www.diabetes.org.uk/guide-to-diabetes/managing-your-diabetes/blood-pressure. *For detailed examples of using the 'teach back' method see the health literacy toolkit at* https://www.hee.nhs.uk/our-work/population-health/training-educational-resources.

DIGITAL LITERACY

Digital literacy is similar to health literacy but may present extra challenges. These include computer skills and having access to technology along with the ability to search, find and use information (Smith & Magnani, 2019). Digital skills are important for interacting with others, accessing services, and doing many jobs. In the UK, the ONS reports that 10% of the population are non-internet users, and in terms of digital skills such as using a search engine and verifying information around 20% of people are lacking in basic digital skills (Office of National Statistics, 2019). Non-users are more likely to be older people. Although these figures may be different post-Covid-19, this still represents a significant number of people who do not have good digital skills.

There is much potential to be gained from digital health interventions and programmes. van Kessel et al. (2022) argue that to gain the full potential of digital media for health and well-being, the skills of digital literacy, health literacy and digital health literacy need to be continuously developed. As with the previous health literacy model shown in Figure 2.9, digital literacy also has levels of functional, interactive, and critical health literacy. However, there is also a need for the ability to rate the 'trustworthiness' of online information. If you go into a health clinic, a health professional may already have selected the appropriate leaflets or booklets to give to you. However, if you search for health topics online a huge array of information is available from across the world. This 'checking' process to validate health information must be done by the person looking for information. This is not just time-consuming but needs analytical skills combined with the ability to decide on the trustworthiness of a source.

MISINFORMATION AND DISINFORMATION

'Misinformation' is false or inaccurate information that may (or may not) cause harm, for example, a rumour. 'Disinformation' is deliberately false or inaccurate information that can spread fear or suspicion, for example, propaganda (UNCHR, 2022). Both can impact people's health behaviours. This can happen through the way information is 'framed' or presented to people as positive or negative. It can also happen electronically through tools that increase certain messages posted on social media such as 'spam-bots' who pretend to be real people or tools that increase the volume of specific messages. Take the example of 'mis' or 'dis' information about vaccines. Messages may encourage belief in something that might not be true and can stop people from getting vaccinated. The now widely disproved link between the Measles, Mumps and Rubella (MMR) vaccine and autism shows how disinformation can affect vaccine uptake, along with some of the global Covid-19 vaccine rumours. Addressing misinformation needs a collaborative approach. To read different countries' actions in this area see the link at the end of the chapter.

SUMMARY

'Developing personal skills' is one of the core health promotion roles that most people associate with health promotion action. Health promotion has the potential to deliver health information and skills through well-planned and designed campaigns. There will always be the appeal of using mass media and information technology, but it cannot be used in isolation. Focussing on one behavioural risk alone ignores the complexities of people's lives and offers little support in addressing the socially determined causes of poor health. Developing personal skills needs to be supported by other areas of the Ottawa Charter. Only then can we create sustainable change that supports the prevention of ill health and the promotion of good health. The next chapter takes us to 'Strengthening community action' where we look outside of individuals and start to explore the communities in which we live.

WIDER READING

ONLINE

If you are interested in the history of health campaigns the National Archives has many of the old films at https://www.nationalarchives.gov.uk/films/view_all_films.htm.

UK Health Days can be found at https://www.nhsemployers.org/events/calendar-national-campaigns. Global World Health Organization (WHO) health days can be found at https://www.who.int/campaigns.

Department for Transport (2022). Enabling behaviour change information pack (in the context of transport), https://www.gov.uk/government/publications/transport-business-case/enabling-behaviour-change-information-pack.

Funke, D., & Flamini, D. (2023). A guide to anti-misinformation actions around the world at https://www.poynter.org/ifcn/anti-misinformation-actions/.

Health Education England's Health literacy toolkit has many examples of ways to improve health literacy at https://www.hee.nhs.uk/our-work/population-health/training-educational-resources.

TEXTBOOKS

Copeman, J., Woodall, J., & Hubley, J. (2021). *Practical health promotion*. Polity Press, Cambridge.

Cook, E., & Wood, L. (2020). *Health psychology: The basics.* Routledge, London.

Corcoran, N. (2013). *Communicating health: Strategies for health promotion.* Sage, London.

Upton, D., & Thirlaway, K. (2014). *Promoting healthy behaviour: A practical guide.* Routledge, London.

Nutbeam, D., Harris, E., & Wise, M. (2022). *Theory in a nutshell.* McGraw-Hill, London.

LISTENING AND WATCHING

'Health Promotion Practice' journal has weekly podcasts about health promotion practice in action available from your podcast provider.

Podcasts cited in this chapter: 'The disability and..' at https://disabilityarts. online/projects/the-disability-and-podcast/ 'Life After Prison' at https:// lifeafterprisonpod.com/ 'Pumping Marvellous' (living with heart failure) at https://pumpingmarvellous.org/.

Current Government campaigns can be found at UK Health Security Agency, for example: How your next bathroom break could save your life, https:// www.youtube.com/watch?v=3oIcKXLhB-k and Don't carry the worry of cancer with you, https://www.youtube.com/watch?v=kDe0PCjtwPg.

ADDITIONAL REFERENCES

These are the additional references this chapter has used where electronic links have not been provided in the chapter.

Ajzen, I. (1991). The theory of planned behaviour. *Organizational Behaviour and Human Decision Processes, 50,* 179–211.

Alexander, S. A., & Shareck, M. (2021). Widening the gap? Unintended consequences of health promotion measures for young people during COVID-19 lockdown. *Health Promotion International, 36*(6), 1783–1794. 10.1093/heapro/daab015.

Ananthapavan, J., Tran, H. N. Q., Morley, B., Hart, E., Kennington, K., Stevens-Cutler, J., Bowe, S. J., Crosland, P., & Moodie, M. (2022). Cost-effectiveness of LiveLighter® – a mass media public education campaign for obesity prevention. *PLoS One, 17*(9), e0274917. 10.1371/journal.pone.0274917.

Bandura, A. (1988). Organizational application of social cognitive theory. *Australian Journal of Management, 13*(2), 275–302.

Becker, M. H. (1974). The health belief model and personal health behaviour. *Health Education Monographs, 2*(4), 324–473.

Carter, S. M., Rychetnik, L., Lloyd, B., Kerridge, I. H., Baur, L., Bauman, A., Hooker, C., & Zask, A. (2011). Evidence, ethics, and values: A framework for health promotion. *Am J Public Health*, *101*(3), 465–472. 10.2105/ajph.2010.195545.

Corcoran, N. (2013). *Communicating health: Strategies for health promotion*. Sage, London.

Crisp, B. R., & Taket, A. (2022). Using a theatre-based programme to prevent gender-based violence: evidence from Australia. *Health Promotion International*. 10.1093/heapro/daac025.

Díaz, D. A., Eckhoff, D. O., Nunes, M., Anderson, M., Keiffer, M., Salazar, I., Knurr, L., Talbert, S., & Duncan, J. B. (2021). Discovery of methods to enhance the care of the LGBTQ+ community. *The Journal for Nurse Practitioners*, *17*(9), 1085–1090. 10.1016/j.nurpra.2021.07.005.

Freebody, P., & Luke, A. (1990). Literacies programs: Debates and demands in cultural context. *Prospect: Australian Journal of E.S.L*, *5*.

Ghahramani, A., de Courten, M., & Prokofieva, M. (2022). The potential of social media in health promotion beyond creating awareness: An integrative review. *BMC Public Health*, *22*(1), 2402. 10.1186/s12889-022-14885-0.

Laverack, G. (2017). The challenge of behaviour change and health promotion. *Challenges*, *8*(2), 25.

Learning and Work Institute. (2022). Mapping skills needs in England. Available at https://learningandwork.org.uk/news-and-policy/literacy-numeracy-england-map/.

Lipsey, A. F., Waterman, A. D., Wood, E. H., & Balliet, W. (2020). Evaluation of first-person storytelling on changing health-related attitudes, knowledge, behaviors, and outcomes: A scoping review. *Patient Educ Couns*, *103*(10), 1922–1934. 10.1016/j.pec.2020.04.014.

Lohr, A. M., Raygoza Tapia, J. P., Valdez, E. S., Hassett, L. C., Gubrium, A. C., Fiddian-Green, A., Larkey, L., Sia, I. G., & Wieland, M. L. (2022). The use of digital stories as a health promotion intervention: A scoping review. *BMC Public Health*, *22*(1), 1180. 10.1186/s12889-022-13595-x.

Michie, S., Atkins, L., & West, R. (2014). The behaviour change wheel. *A guide to designing interventions*. 1st ed. Silverback Publishing, UK.

Mwaba, K., Senyurek, G., Ulman, Y. I., Minckas, N., Hughes, P., Paphitis, S., Andrabi, S., Ben Salem, L., Ahmad, L., Ahmad, A., & Mannell, J. (2021). 'My story is like a magic wand': A qualitative study of personal storytelling and activism to stop violence against women in Turkey. *Glob Health Action*, *14*(1), 1927331. 10.1080/16549716.2021.1927331.

National Literacy Trust. (2023). The importance of literacy. Available at https://literacytrust.org.uk/information/what-is-literacy/.

Nutbeam, D. (2000). Health literacy as a public health goal: A challenge for contemporary health education and communication strategies into the 21st century. *Health Promotion International*, *15*(3), 259–267. 10.1093/heapro/15.3.259.

Nutbeam, D., & Lloyd, J. E. (2021). Understanding and responding to health literacy as a social determinant of health. *Annual Reviews of Public Health*, *42*, 159–173. 10.1146/annurev-publhealth-090419-102529.

Office for Health Improvement and Disparities. (2022). Nicotine vaping in England: 2022 evidence update main findings. Available at https://www.gov. uk/government/publications/nicotine-vaping-in-england-2022-evidence-update/nicotine-vaping-in-england-2022-evidence-update-main-findings.

Office of National Statistics. (2019). Exploring the UK's digital divide. Available at https://www.ons.gov.uk/peoplepopulationandcommunity/householdcharacteristics/homeinternetandsocialmediausage/articles/exploringtheuksdigitaldivide/2019-03-04.

Office of National Statistics. (2021). Adult smoking habits in the UK: 2021. Available at https://www.ons.gov.uk/peoplepopulationandcommunity/healthandsocialcare/healthandlifeexpectancies/bulletins/adultsmokinghabitsingreatbritain/2021#:~:text=In%202021%2C%2015.1%25%20of%20men, lowest%20(8.0%25)%20in%202021.

Pehere, N. K., & Yadavalli, S. (2021). Using street plays as a populist way to spread eye health awareness: An experience. *Indian Journal of Ophthalmology*, *69*(5). https://journals.lww.com/ijo/Fulltext/2021/05000/Using_street_plays_as_a_populist_way_to_spread_eye.61.aspx.

Prochaska, J. O., & Diclemente, C. C. (1983). Stages and processes of self-change in smoking: towards an integrative model fo change. *Journal of Consulting and Clinical Psychology*, *51*(3), 390–395.

Public Health England. (2021). Relaunch of the Act FAST campaign to improve stroke outcomes. Available at https://www.gov.uk/government/news/relaunch-of-the-act-fast-campaign-to-improve-stroke-outcomes.

Scottish Government. (2022). Naloxone provision. Available at https://www. gov.scot/policies/alcohol-and-drugs/naloxone-provision/.

Smith, B., & Magnani, J. W. (2019). New technologies, new disparities: The intersection of electronic health and digital health literacy. *Int J Cardiol*, *292*, 280–282. 10.1016/j.ijcard.2019.05.066.

Stellefson, M., Paige, S. R., Chaney, B. H., & Chaney, J. D. (2020). Evolving role of social media in health promotion: Updated responsibilities for health education specialists. *International Journal of Environmental Research in Public Health*, *17*(4). 10.3390/ijerph17041153.

UK Government. (2022). Prison education: a review of reading education in prisons. Available at https://www.gov.uk/government/publications/prison-education-a-review-of-reading-education-in-prisons/prison-education-a-re-view-of-reading-education-in-prisons.

UNCHR. (2022). Factsheet 4: Types of misinformation and disinformation. Available at https://unhcr.org/innovation/wp-content/uploads/2022/02/Factsheet-4.pdf.

van Kessel, R., Wong, B. L. H., Clemens, T., & Brand, H. (2022). Digital health literacy as a super determinant of health: More than simply the sum of its parts. *Internet Interventions, 27,* 100500. 10.1016/j.invent.2022.100500.

Wang, C. C., Yi, W. K., Tao, Z. W., & Carovano, K. (1998). Photovoice as a participatory health promotion strategy. *Health Promotion International, 13*(1), 75–86. (Health Promotion International).

West, R., Michie, S., Rubin, G. J., & Amlôt, R. (2020). Applying principles of behaviour change to reduce SARS-CoV-2 transmission. *Nature Human Behaviour, 4*(5), 451–459. 10.1038/s41562-020-0887-9.

World Health Organization. (2022). Health literacy development for the prevention and control of noncommunicable diseases: Volume 4. Case studies from WHO National Health Literacy Demonstration Projects. Available at https://www.who.int/publications/i/item/9789240055391.

World Stroke Organization. (2023). Signs of stroke FAST. Available at https://www.world-stroke.org/world-stroke-day-campaign/why-stroke-matters/stroke-treatment/signs-of-stroke-fast.

3

STRENGTHENING COMMUNITY ACTION

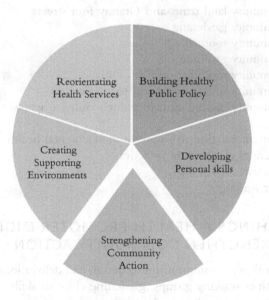

Figure 3.1 Strengthening community action.

DOI: 10.4324/9781003462323-4

- Five things a health promoter might do to strengthen community action
- Overview
- Why community action?
- Social participation
- Community engagement
- Social capital
- Four community-centred approaches
- Time banking
- Peer support
- Citizen science
- Building capacity
- Power and empowerment
- Co-production
- Asset-based approaches
- The Wigan deal
- Community-led housing
- Community land trusts and Granby four streets
- Community gardening
- Community football
- Community profiling
- Community mobilisation
- Community mobilisation and road safety
- Community mobilisation to reduce violence against women and girls
- Community action to improve men's mental health.
- Challenges of community action
- Summary
- Wider reading

FIVE THINGS A HEALTH PROMOTER MIGHT DO TO STRENGTHEN COMMUNITY ACTION

(1) Work with communities to design and deliver local initiatives such as walking groups, gardening clubs or skills classes.

(2) Set up and facilitate peer education or peer support groups or cafes.

(3)   Promote volunteering opportunities, skill exchanges or ex-
      isting community projects.
(4)   Be part of, or support, community co-operatives to regenerate
      spaces, houses or streets.
(5)   Get involved with citizen science or community advocacy
      (Figure 3.1).

OVERVIEW

Community action is about communities taking action to improve
their health using the assets and resources that they have available to
them. A community is a 'group of people joined together by a
common interest, characteristic or experience' (Buck et al., 2021).
Sometimes we refer to people living in communities as 'citizens'. A
community is not just a geographical place. Goodman et al. (2014)
suggest that the term community refers to both people and places
and could be:

• People who share a common connection or do something
  together like a faith group.
• A venue linked with key activities like education or work.
• An area that is physically defined, geographically defined, culturally
  defined or administratively defined. For example a housing estate,
  a village or shared characteristics like an ethnic group.

These definitions overlap but everyone is part of a community, and
often more than one different type. For example, you might go to a
place of worship, belong to a workplace, attend a community group
and live in a town. You can reflect on the communities you belong
to in activity 3a.

WHY COMMUNITY ACTION?

Our health is connected to where we live. Features of communities
such as the clubs, services or shops, the housing, the local parks, the
public transport links or the physical location all influence the health
of people living in communities. Many organisations are working in
communities already. Perhaps you even belong to one? For example,

in the UK, the Ramblers UK runs local well-being walks https://www.ramblers.org.uk/, the Women's Institute (WI) runs local women's groups https://www.thewi.org.uk/, The u3a runs learning and staying active groups for people no longer in work https://www.u3a.org.uk/, and The Scouts Association https://www.scouts.org.uk/ offers life skills for young people. There are also community choirs, faith groups, exercise classes, gardening clubs, playgroups, youth clubs, and social clubs … the list is endless.

Practitioner skills activity 3a: Community health and well-being.

Think about the community in which you live. How would you define your community? What services and resources are there that might help to promote physical, social, spiritual or mental health and well-being? How would you find out about your community and who lives in it? What groups already work in your community?

'Connected communities that act and take control are healthier communities' (p. 5) (McGregor-Paterson, 2021). Communities are more likely to come together around issues that matter to them. Covid-19 lockdowns saw a wide range of ways that communities tried to unite and self-organise, across the UK (and in other countries) to support each other in difficult times. Community cooking, collecting medication for neighbours, or outdoor 'in your own garden' street events are just a few examples.

National Institute of Clinical Excellence (2017) states that initiatives developed in partnership with communities are better able to address local needs and thus mean more to the people living in those areas. Community action is also an important part of achieving the SDGs. For example, SDG 2 'zero hunger' needs community food initiatives and SDG 5 'gender equality' needs everyone to challenge behaviours that jeopardise women's safety. An example of a food initiative is given below.

Health promotion in practice example: Foodcycle (UK).

Foodcycle is a charity active across England and South Wales. It aims to connect communities, inspire change and support mental well-being by ensuring those who are hungry are nourished. It uses a community dining model where volunteers use surplus food to provide meals for people living in local communities. The community dining model, not only supports eliminating hunger but provides company for those who are lonely. Read more at www.foodcycle.org.uk.

Community action makes use of physical assets or resources such as leisure centres. It supports the transformation of spaces, for example from derelict or neglected to vibrant and useful. This type of action promotes 'community resilience'. This is a term that means communities are stronger and work together more, and thus better prepared in adverse times.

Effective action involves people doing things for themselves, rather than having things done to them. For example, when a council decides to change a bus route or close a library without consulting the community first, this is an example of something being 'done' to a community. When communities plan their actions such as street closures for parties, organising litter picks or community fundraising events, they are taking action for themselves. The radio station example below shows an example of community involvement.

Health promotion in practice example: Community radio stations in England.

Examples of UK community-based radio stations are All.fm in Manchester (England) https://allfm.org/ and Vectis radio based on the Isle of Wight (England) https://www.vectisradio.com/. Vectis Radio also runs a 4Ps project which is a radio training school aimed at young people and disadvantaged adults on the Isle of Wight. 'Reprezent' is a community radio station exclusively for young people in London (England) at https://www.reprezent.org.uk/. Radio Regan is a charity that has set up community radio stations and trained people from disadvantaged communities in the North West of England to be part of community radio. Their website tells you more at http://www.communityradiotoolkit.net/health/health-radio/.

SOCIAL PARTICIPATION

Social participation is the ability of a person to engage within the society or communities in which they live. People can be excluded from society in different ways. For example, someone who is unemployed may have fewer connections and is less able to participate in social activities. Communities have an important role to play in increasing social participation. For example, an initiative to support people back into work is 'working wardrobe' (Manchester, England), which provides people with suits for interviews. Read more at https://www.gmworkingwardrobe.co.uk/. An example of older people and social participation is given in the health promotion in practice example below.

Health promotion in practice example: Age UK and participation of older people.

Age UK is an older person charity that encourages the social participation of older people in society. They work to raise awareness of the issues faced by older people. 'Meet Fred' is a video designed to highlight the 1.2 million older people experiencing loneliness. You can watch this at https://www.youtube.com/watch?v=Q4fo0XXiTG0&feature=emb_imp_woyt. *Age UK's community-based services include befriending schemes, lunch clubs, handyperson services, and help with shopping and wellness services such as foot care and exercise classes. They even have a 'cat café'* https://www.ageuk.org.uk/discover/2019/december/cat-cafe/. *As a charity organisation Age UK has events and activities in communities across the UK. Explore their website for more actions at* https://www.ageuk.org.uk/.

Douglas et al. (2017) explore three types of social participation.

- **Social connections.** This is connections with other people.
- **Informal social participation.** The activities that people engage in such as social activities.
- **Volunteering.** These are activities that benefit others, usually for a specific purpose.

All three types of social participation can influence health and those who are more able to participate tend to report better health. Action in communities can focus on one type of social participation like building social connections, for example, Friendship benches. These are community benches that you sit on as an invitation for people to come and talk to you. A Canadian example for young people aimed at improving mental health can be found at https://thefriendshipbench.org/. Other actions can include all three areas such as 'Repair Cafes' in the below example.

Health promotion in practice example: Repair cafés.

Repair cafes are locations or pop-up events where local communities can bring broken household items such as furniture or household electronics to be repaired by volunteers. It aims to reduce waste, share skills and promote a repair culture. It is also a way to connect residents to each other who may not usually know each other. Read more from a Welsh example at www.repair.cafewales.org. *Repair Café International shows a list of repair cafés from all over the world, as well as tips on how to repair items like furniture and electronics at* https://www.repaircafe.org/en/.

COMMUNITY ENGAGEMENT

The World Health Organization (2022) calls community engagement, the 'glue' that unites communities. Corbin et al. (2021) state that the question is not whether communities should be engaged in their health, but how. He says strategies to strengthen community engagement are vital, especially as emergencies such as Covid-19 mean traditional community engagement strategies like community meetings are not viable. The author suggests the following for more successful engagement:

- Accessible information for everyone.
- The use of multiple communication channels.
- Involvement of key community leaders.
- The use of existing community relationships or infrastructures.
- Recognition of barriers such as mistrust.

Health promoters use strategies like these to build community engagement. They work with people and use existing spaces like community halls to work with communities. If we cannot engage people in action, then efforts to reduce pandemics like Covid-19 or to reduce threats to health through climate change will not work. Take the example of SDG 15 'life on land'. This goal focuses on protecting habitats and biodiversity, halting deforestation and advancing conservation. These efforts involve everyone. For example, tree planting projects need volunteers to support the huge amount of re-planting work that needs to be done. One person cannot do this by themselves. An example of the importance of community engagement for 'Avian influenza' is given below.

Health promotion in practice example: Avian influenza (UK).

Avian influenza (bird flu) is a global disease. At the time of writing this book (2023), the virus is circulating through the bird population in the UK and is the world's largest-ever outbreak. Responses to this are targeted at communities of birdkeepers, farmers and the general public to engage in prevention strategies to reduce the spread of Avian influenza. Action includes maintaining good biosecurity (for example fencing birds to keep them apart from wildlife), registering poultry, signing up for alerts, restricting poultry gatherings and reporting dead or sick birds to the Department for Environment, Food and Rural Affairs (Defra) in England and Wales and the Animal and Plant Health Agency (APHA) in Scotland. Engaging communities that keep birds is essential to limit the spread of avian influenza. Read more at https:// www.gov.uk/guidance/avian-influenza-bird-flu.

SOCIAL CAPITAL

Practitioner skills activity 3b: Could you borrow a cup of sugar?

Imagine you are making a cake and you have run out of sugar. The shops are closed. Could you go to any of the neighbours in your street and ask them if you could borrow some sugar? If you think yes, your neighbours would lend you some sugar, then this is an example of 'high social capital', and if you said no, this is an example of 'low social capital'. Those people who have higher social capital usually have people that they can talk to nearby and can call on in a time of need.

Social capital is the links that people form within their communities and the value that these networks bring. Social relationships are a resource, and having positive relationships can build social capital. The practitioner skills activity 3b gives an example of social capital. There are three different types of social capital illustrated in Figure 3.2. These are bridging social capital, bonding social capital and linking social capital.

Practitioner skills activity 3c: Definitions of social capital.

Match the definitions to one of the three types of social capital in Figure 3.2. For example, working with local businesses to encourage better recycling schemes would match 'linking' social capital. As there is an overlap between the types of social capital, decide which one fits best.

- *Going on a family picnic.*
- *Parents in a school learning alongside skills with other parents to create healthy lunchbox meals.*
- *Publicising local community groups like craft clubs and playgroups through local businesses.*

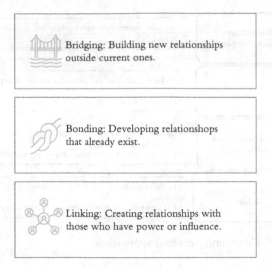

Figure 3.2 Different types of social capital.

Participating in community projects and initiatives can change people. For example, a Men's Health Project in Dublin (Ireland) notes the importance of community engagement and capacity building to both promote men's health and encourage participation. In addition, men reported a transfer of skills outside the project, for example gaining leadership skills that can be used in other areas of their lives (Lefkowich et al., 2017). See a later section in the chapter for more on men's health.

FOUR COMMUNITY-CENTRED APPROACHES

Traditional approaches to community development have been split into 'top-down' or 'bottom-up' approaches. Peters et al. (2022) suggest a top-down approach is a 'deficit' model that sees communities only as service receivers or the community is talked about as a 'problem' to be fixed. A bottom-up approach recognises the strength of communities. A bottom-up approach is a preferred way of working in health promotion as it recognises and builds on existing skills and capacity and other assets in the community. See Chapter 2 'Developing personal Skills' for a bottom-up communication model.

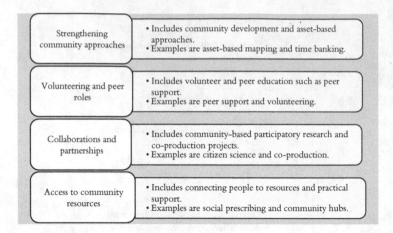

Figure 3.3 Community-centred approaches.

There are a wide variety of ways that change can happen in communities. National UK guidance divides community-centred approaches into four strands (Office for Health Improvement and Disparities, 2022). Figure 3.3 shows the four strands.

Examples of three approaches in Figure 3.3. are discussed in more detail below: time banking, peer support groups and citizen science. Social prescribing is included in Chapter 6 'Reorientating health services'.

TIME BANKING

Time banking is a not-for-monetary-profit approach that uses the idea of 'exchange'. A person gives one hour, and they get something back in return. It is a way of sharing skills, meeting new people and feeling more connected to others in a community. The idea is built on using people with one type of skill to support the unmet needs of people who have different skills. For example, a person might do two hours of gardening for someone, and get a shirt mended in return. Modern-time banking follows five core values that are linked to Edgar Cahn who conceptualised modern-time banking in America. Figure 3.4 shows the five characteristics of time banking.

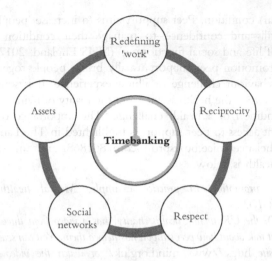

Figure 3.4 Characteristics of time banking.

The five characteristics of time banking in Figure 3.4 are:

- Assets: everyone has something of value to share.
- Redefining work: not all work needs to have a monetary currency exchange.
- Reciprocity: helping people is a two-way process.
- Social networks: sharing can strengthen social capital (see the section on social capital in this chapter).
- Respect: recognises anyone can participate and everyone is valued.

Websites such as Time Banking UK https://timebanking.org/ and Timebanks.org https://www.timebanks.org/ in the USA have more information and case studies to read.

PEER SUPPORT

Peer support is a way for people to give, or gain, support from others who might be in a similar situation. For example, people living with a long-term condition offer support to other people with the same (or similar) condition. Peer support aims to increase 'people's knowledge, skills and confidence to manage their condition improving quality of life and social functioning' (NHS England, 2017) (p. 5). In health promotion peer support usually brings people together with a shared behaviour challenge or illness experience. It is sometimes the bridge between the health service and the reality of living with a long-term condition or a health challenge. The importance of child and adolescent access to peer support is highlighted in The Lancet podcast https://thelancetvoice.buzzsprout.com/861868 and an example of mental health is below.

Health promotion in practice example: Mental health and peer support (UK).

MIND, the UK mental health charity, has a video from three peer support groups that talk about how peer support has helped them. You can search for this on their website https://www.mind.org.uk/ *or watch the video at this link* https://www.mind.org.uk/information-support/drugs-and-treatments/peer-support/about-peer-support/ *(MIND, 2022). The Mental Health Foundation provides a range of resources around the different types of peer support and where to get support at* https://www.mentalhealth.org.uk/explore-mental-health/a-z-topics/peer-support.

Breastfeeding is an area that has shown good evidence for peer support. The WHO-UNICEF Global Breastfeeding Collective recognises the need to advocate for breastfeeding including improving access to skilled breastfeeding counselling in health facilities and communities {WHO and UNICEF, 2019). Read more at https://www.globalbreastfeedingcollective.org/. In the UK, NICE guidance (2014) recommends that service providers provide breastfeeding peer support programmes alongside other services, and evidence shows that community-based peer support programmes can promote the early initiation of breastfeeding (Shakya et al., 2017). Breastfeeding cafes for example are set up to bring people together through breastfeeding. For an example see Lowestoft and Waveney cafes (England) at https://www.lowestoftandwaveneybreastfeeding.co.uk/breastfeeding-cafes. Peer support can also be delivered online through mechanisms like social media. Facebook breastfeeding support groups are widely used in the UK, and research suggest they are valued locally for their connections to face-to-face local services, as well as other mothers (Morse & Brown, 2021).

Practitioner skills activity 3d: Peer support.
How do you think peer support groups could work to support those living with a long-term health condition like diabetes or stroke? Look on the peer support pages of Diabetes UK https://www.diabetes.org.uk/how_we_help/local_support_groups/peer-support *or the Stroke Association which has a video about stroke survivors' support groups* https://www.stroke.org.uk/finding-support/stroke-support-groups.

CITIZEN SCIENCE

A citizen is a word used to describe residents or inhabitants of a place. Citizen science is a participatory research method that aims to engage volunteers in activities, such as collecting data or data analysis. Citizens may have some or no research training or experience. Projects include:

- Measuring air quality, plant monitoring and national pollinator schemes. See more and join in at https://www.ceh.ac.uk/data/web-based-apps (UK Centre for Ecology and Hydrology, 2022).
- Health projects such as physical activity and nutrition (see the health promotion in practice example below).
- Global projects that can be done from anywhere in the world. Read more and join in at https://www.zooniverse.org/projects. Project areas include medicine, the arts, climate, nature, social science, space, literature, language and history.
- Citizen puzzles and games. For example, Cancer Research UK has used puzzles and activities to support research into four cancer types. See more at https://www.cancerresearchuk.org/get-involved/citizen-science/the-projects. You can also see https://citizensciencegames.com/ which has games to help researchers with areas like memory and Covid-19.

Citizen science uses different levels of participation. Projects can be 'contributory style projects' where people collect data. They can also be 'collaborative' projects, where people participate or co-design elements of a project. They can also be 'citizen-led' projects where citizens are involved in the whole project. Marks et al. (2022) suggest increasing the different types of people involved and expanding projects to include health equity topics. See an example of a food environment project in health promotion in practice example below.

Health promotion in practice example: Exploring the food environment in Canada.

The Local Environmental Action on Food (LEAF) project is a community-based intervention in 17 communities in Alberta, Canada. It uses citizen science to engage residents in monitoring and acting on local food environments (physical, communication, economic, social and political) and nutrition policies for children and young people. It is a collaborative project between a research team, the healthcare delivery system, communities and individuals. Communities collect data through an online data collection tool about the food environment in which they live and recommendations are developed from the findings. See more at (Aylward et al., 2022).

BUILDING CAPACITY

Involving communities in their health may not be easy to do. For example, how do you bring people together of different backgrounds? How do you encourage action with people who are not used to being asked what they want, or do not feel they have anything to offer? The idea of taking ownership of a project might be overwhelming for many people. The health promotion in practice example below explores what they did in projects in the Philippines.

Health promotion in practice example: Developing community leadership in the Philippines.

Outreach International works in several low-income countries to reduce poverty using a community-led approach. In the Philippines, they recognised that managing projects such as community water systems or microloans are complex and technical, especially as many participants do not have much schooling after primary school. The organisation provided 'on the job' training on planning, implementation and management of projects. Training also includes skills in fundraising, writing proposals, and establishing relationships with local government agencies. The aim is that people in the community go on to be community leaders and communities take ownership of the projects. Read more on community leadership in the Philippines at Cloete & Dasig Salazar (2022). See more on Outreach International and its projects such as rice loans, irrigation systems and eco stoves at https://outreach-international.org/our-work/approach/.

- People from Black, Asian and Minority ethnic (BAME) groups
- People from LGBTQ+ communities
- People who communicate differently
- People with dementia
- Older people who need a high level of support
- People who are not affiliated to any organised group or community
- The location in which people live i.e. homeless, care homes or prisons

Figure 3.5 Groups at risk of being excluded.

The idea of building capacity is that everyone can be involved in community projects and that all community members can build their skills, knowledge and experience to support action. The Social Care Institute for Excellence (2022) lists the communities traditionally excluded from community projects. These are shown in Figure 3.5.

Figure 3.5 includes groups who communicate differently such as those having English as a second language, or those using sign language. It also includes those who might have a cognitive impairment (actual or assumed), groups who have a history of exclusion, groups who are excluded based on where they live or groups who rely on others such as those with a carer.

For sustained engagement in community action, everyone needs to have the opportunity to be involved or to be represented. Even when we think we have done this, there may still be people missing. Take the example of schools. Important work is done in schools to support children's health and well-being but how do we include children who are excluded from school or who find attending difficult? See practitioner skills activity 3e to think more about groups at risk of exclusion. Building capacity means finding different ways that people can be involved in the action.

Practitioner skills activity 3e: Communicating differently.

Look at Figure 3.5. Choose one of the groups at risk of exclusion. Why do you think they might be excluded from community projects or actions? What could you do to reach out to people living in these communities and encourage participation?

POWER AND EMPOWERMENT

A major barrier to achieving meaningful and sustainable change is power. The declaration of Alma Ata (World Health Organization, 1978) states that people have the right and duty to participate individually and collectively in the planning and implementation of their healthcare. However, not everyone can participate equally in decisions about their health. This is not just about access to healthcare and available healthcare services. This is also about what is happening in and around the communities in which people live. Having decent, affordable housing, reliable transport networks, and being able to participate in well-paid work influences health and well-being. Healthier communities tend to have more 'power' and assets available to them. Power is central to health and the systems that influence health and well-being. We see the power in our daily interactions for example at work, in education or in healthcare. Look at activity 3f for an example of power in healthcare. Power shapes 'actions, processes and outcomes' (Sriram et al., 2018) and this means it can exclude people and stop people from participating in taking action or being involved in their communities.

Practitioner skills activity 3f: Power and empowerment.

Think about the last time you went to see someone about your health, like a doctor, optician, physiotherapist, pharmacist or dentist. Who was holding the power? What was the power relationship like? We you able to participate in the conversation equally? Were you able to express what you wanted? Do you think your age, gender, education or ethnicity impacted your ability to participate in the conversation?

Empowerment and power are complex areas and are still much debated. It is generally agreed that empowerment is a good thing, which can lead to better equity, and better health outcomes and allow people to increase control over their lives (Popay et al., 2021). See the example below about 'The Parks Community' which supports community action. Different types of empowerment can lead to positive impacts. For example, a study in Glasgow explored empowerment through a regeneration project. They measured individual empowerment (through housing development), and collective empowerment (through neighbourhood regeneration) and found that both types of empowerment, (particularly proactive forms such as influencing decisions) were associated with mental well-being (Kearns & Whitley, 2020).

There is no agreed definition of empowerment. One way to conceptualise empowerment is to think of power a little like 'assets'. Educational empowerment such as formal education (going to school or college) can bring better employment opportunities and self-confidence. Community empowerment is centred around cultural, and social values or feelings of belonging to a community. Employment empowerment is having a meaningful job, where employees have autonomy and control over the ways they work. Economic empowerment is having financial power, directly (having money) or indirectly through community economic growth.

Health promotion in practice example: The Parks Community (UK).

The park's website is an online knowledge hub and network for groups who are 'friends of parks' or 'green spaces'. Case studies come from across England showing what local park uses can achieve. They include guides on how to host meetings and events as well as how to campaign for action, improve relationships with service users, and manage plans and ways to save green space. You can read more at https://parkscommunity.org.uk/.

Community action should try and remove or reduce traditional forms of power, such as those in charge like local councils making all the decisions. If people are going to be empowered, it means other people have to give up that power. This process is called 'empowerment'. However, empowerment is more than just talking to people or educating them about health behaviours. It is a process or social change (and sometimes political change) that transfers ownership of action to communities.

An example of how communities can take ownership of assets comes from Scotland. Scotland has a policy that enables the 'asset transfer' of resources back to communities. This allows communities to take control over physical assets in their communities like buildings or community spaces. You can read more at https://dtascommunityownership.org.uk/. It can take many years, but ways that health promoters can work to empower others are building an evidence base and will form the basis for health promotion activities in the future. There is some wider reading around this area at the end of the chapter.

CO-PRODUCTION

Co-production is an equal relationship between people who use services, and the people who design and deliver services (Think Local Act Personal, 2021). This is based on the principle that those who use a service are the best people to help design it. For example, most health services are designed by people who are not unwell and will not be using them and most new housing developments are designed by people who won't live there.

The concept of co-production starts with an idea that everyone in a community is involved in a shared vision of what needs to change and everyone is involved in generating collective solutions. A ladder of co-production has been created to show the steps towards the full co-production process, with each step up the ladder being a step towards meaningful co-production. See Figure 3.6. The ladder of co-production.

Figure 3.6 shows the ladder of co-production. The ladder is used to help organisations and the people working in them identify ways to move up the ladder. The steps are described below.

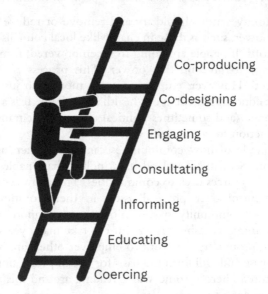

Figure 3.6 The ladder of co-production.

- Coercion: People are told about changes that will happen to them and their views are not taken into account. This is an example of 'top down' as discussed earlier.
- Education: People using the services are told about them.
- Informing: People are given information about services, and why these decisions have been made.
- Consulting: Asking people their opinions about services, although this may not result in a change to a service.
- Engagement: Asking people for their opinions and including these views in the service design and delivery.
- Co-design: Including people and their views and experiences in the service design or delivery but not in everything.
- Co-production: An equal relationship between the people using services and the people designing and delivering services including how they can best meet the needs of the people using them.

More about the ladder of co-production can be found at the 'Think Local Act Personal' website which has videos and podcasts about co-production available at https://www.thinklocalactpersonal.org.uk/Browse/Co-production/ with videos at https://www.youtube.com/watch?v=kEgsJXLo7M8.

ASSET-BASED APPROACHES

An old African Igbo and Yoruba proverb says, '*It takes a village to raise a child*', meaning everyone should be involved in 'raising a child', but what does it take to raise a village? The answer is that it takes the whole village. This is really what the essence of 'asset based' approaches are, as they focus on building strengths of an entire 'village', or community. The community are the one who create and invest in change, using whatever resources are available as a starting point; for example, natural spaces, cultural bonds, buildings and people (Nel, 2018). The idea behind asset-based approaches is that organisations outside of the community, no matter how well-meaning, can unintentionally emphasise problems. This means 'needs' are then addressed from a 'problem' perspective and the community may become dependent on others, rather than creating solutions themselves. This approach is sometimes framed as a 'deficit' approach as the focus is on what is wrong with a community.

An asset-based approach turns this idea around, and instead asks, what resources and strengths communities already have. How can the 'village' build a community? And how can the village solve problems or stop problems before they start? The positive things that a community has are 'assets'. Many people think of assets as physical things, such as a leisure centre or library but there are other types of assets as well. Public Health England (2018) suggests four categories of assets. These are shown with examples in Figure 3.7.

Using Figure 3.7 as a guide these are examples of different categories of assets.

- Skills and knowledge: A community might have people who are skilled in a wide variety of areas such as carpentry, gardening, different languages, cooking or caring for children.
- Resources and facilities: There could be a college or library with community space available.
- Friends, neighbours and groups: People may all know each other in that community and there could be a variety of groups and activities happening.
- Physical, environmental and economic: There could be physical resources such as green spaces, blue spaces (the sea or river), parks or a leisure centre.

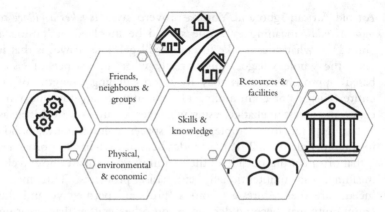

Figure 3.7 Four categories of assets.

Identifying the assets that exist in a community is important, as this can ensure that everyone knows what is available already and that everyone can access these assests. For health promoters working in a community, it is a way of recognising that all communities have strengths, it stops duplication of work and allows for better use of resources. It also reminds us that every community has assets that can be used directly, or as a platform to promote health and well-being.

Practitioner skills activity 3g: Community assets in a local area.

Find out the assets in your community. Look online at the community in which you live. Try searching for 'what's on', or 'community groups' and the name of your community. Is there a social media page for your community? Look at your local council website. You could also take a bus or walk around your community and see what opportunities or assets it has.

THE WIGAN DEAL

In 2010 local councils in England needed to make big financial savings in response to large funding cuts from the Government. This meant big changes to public services in areas like education and social care. In Wigan, in Greater Manchester (England), the council sought to change the way public services were delivered through an asset-based way of working. This meant changing the way public services were designed and delivered and working with local people through leadership and a commitment to long-term change. The outcome of this process was an informal agreement between the people that live and work in Wigan and the local council. This is known as 'the Wigan deal'.

The Wigan deal is split into two parts; what the council will do and what those who live and work in the borough will do. For example, the council says it will support the local economy to grow, create opportunities for young people and keep council tax low. The community says it will recycle more, support local businesses and help protect children and the vulnerable. You can watch a short animation video on the Wigan deal (Wigan Council, 2018) at https://www. wigan.gov.uk/Council/The-Deal/The-Deal.aspx. A video that shows how relationships between the council and residents are available here https://www.kingsfund.org.uk/publications/wigan-deal. Both are also available on YouTube by searching 'Wigan deal'.

COMMUNITY LED-HOUSING

Housing can have a major impact on health as outlined in Chapter 1 'The field of health promotion'. Community-led housing is an umbrella term for housing initiatives run by groups of people who want to build homes in the communities in which they live. It includes people coming together to help to build, renovate or repurpose existing houses or spaces. This might be intergenerational housing (grandparent-parent-children) in one space or co-operatives who work together to create housing projects. The best way to understand community-led housing projects is to explore some of the case studies on websites. The website for Community Led Housing London (Community Led Housing London, 2022) has different examples of community-led housing projects including co-housing where a group of residents design housing to create communal spaces, for example, laundry rooms, kitchens or gardens. See https://www.communityledhousing. london/projects/. In Scotland, the Communities Housing Trust (Communities Housing Trust, 2022) also has a range of case studies and multiple videos to watch https://www.chtrust.co.uk/case-studies1. html. There are also housing co-operatives for students. Read more at https://www.students.coop/.

COMMUNITY LAND TRUSTS AND GRANBY FOUR STREETS

Community land trusts are democratic, non-profit organisations that own and develop land for the benefit of the community (Community Land Trust Network, 2022). Granby Four Streets Community Land Trust (in Liverpool, England) is an area of four streets in Liverpool. In 2010, residents came together to try and improve housing in disrepair and enhance the four streets. The community land trust has created a community garden project and a winter garden indoor space and bought and renovated housing. You can read more about the project at https://www.granby4streetsclt. co.uk/. There is also a podcast on The Guardian website about how Granby Four Streets came about https://www.theguardian.com/ politics/commentisfree/audio/2018/feb/14/the-alternatives-how-liverpool-suburb-upended-housing-market-podcast.

COMMUNITY GARDENING

Community gardening benefits have been reported historically and today. Community gardening offers individual and collective benefits ranging from food security and social connections to social resilience (Joshi & Wende, 2022). Globally, they have also been reported to create jobs, act as an educational exchange, and support communities to be more climate resilient (International Fund for Agricultural Development, 2023). A community garden is a space where people come together to cultivate or 'garden' land. How this is done varies considerably, for example, Tŷ Pawb in Wrexham (Wales) as part of their arts and cultural community space have a community garden converted from an old car park. See more at https://www.typawb.wales/about/.

Globally, community gardening is organised in different ways. For example in Seattle (USA), 'P-patch community gardening' schemes are similar to community allotment schemes. Read and watch more at this link https://www.seattle.gov/neighborhoods/p-patch-gardening. In Australia Truong et al. (2022) highlight 'community greening' outreach work, where social housing estates that traditionally have less access to green space are enhanced through community growing approaches. You can read, listen and watch more about the Royal Botanical Gardens in Sydney and their 'Branch out: growing communities with gardens programme' and community greening programme at https://www.rbgsyd.nsw.gov.au/learn/community-greening.

Health promotion in practice example: Starting a community garden (UK).
Some organisations offer support in creating a community garden. The Royal Horticultural Society (RHS) 2023 has a campaign called the 'big seed sow' as a way of bringing people together for a nationwide week of action to share seeds and sow seeds together. You can see more at https://www.rhs.org.uk/get-involved/big-seed-sow. *The Eden Project has a guide on starting a community garden project at* https://www.edenprojectcommunities.com/stuff-to-do/plant-community-garden *as do councils in the UK, for example, Lewisham's guide to creating a community garden (London, UK) at* https://lewisham.gov.uk/myservices/environment/allotments/community-gardens.

COMMUNITY FOOTBALL

Sports can be so much more than physical activity, and community activities involving football can be found across the world. Football is 'a perfect vehicle that transcends race, religion, language and gender to bring about a change' (Slum soccer, 2023). In the UK, football has been used as a way to engage a wide variety of learners in schools across the curriculum, not just in physical education classes, but in areas like literacy and numeracy. The Scottish Football Association's 'Learning through Football' website gives examples of how football can be integrated into classroom learning at https://learningthroughfootball.scottishfa.co.uk/.

Outside of the classroom is where we can see the many exciting ways football can be used for health promotion and health education community action. 'Slum Soccer India' is an organisation that aims to bring about social change in those living in slums. Their projects aim to increase life skills and improve education outcomes. For example, 'Edukick' and 'model city Delhi' promote gender equality, health and sanitation. Read more at https://slumsoccer.org/. 'Tackle Africa' is an organisation based in East, West and South Africa that aims to educate young people on sexual health through football. For example, football drills are associated with sexual health messages. Read more at https://tackleafrica.org/. 'Grassroots Soccer' runs over 40 countries in Africa, South America, Asia and the Caribbean. It focuses on promoting adolescent health through football giving young people health information, skills and access to health services to empower young people. Read more at https://grassrootsoccer.org/. ISF Cambodia uses both education and football in economically deprived communities in Cambodia. Read more about their community development work in education and their provision of grassroots football at https://isfcambodia.org/.

COMMUNITY PROFILING

A community profile is a way of building up a picture of a community. It is used to identify past influences, and present conditions and make future predictions about the health of the community. It maps physical, social, environmental, and economic conditions using available quantitative data, such as statistics and this is sometimes supplemented with qualitative data, such as interviews with community leaders. Data is usually collected on the makeup of a community such as age, gender, ethnicity and health status alongside data on housing, employment, education, crime, environment and access to services.

In the UK, Indices of Deprivation are a useful tool in this process. This is an official measure of relative deprivation for small areas such as postcodes, boroughs or towns. In England, the English Indices of Deprivation (Department for Levelling Up, 2019) show data for areas such as housing, education, income and employment at the postcode level. Wales uses a similar tool, the Welsh Index of Multiple Deprivation (WIMD) (Welsh Government, 2019), Scotland, the Scottish Index of Multiple Deprivation (SMID) (Scottish Government), Northern Ireland, the Northern Ireland Multiple Deprivation Measure (Northern Ireland Statistics Research Agency, 2017). All resources are interactive, and you can look up individual postcodes or areas. See the practitioner skills activity below for more on community profiling.

Practitioner skills activity 3h: Community profiling.

Several resources give you basic information about the area where you live that can be used for a community profile. These include population or census data https://www.ons.gov.uk/census *and commercial websites such as* https://www.streetcheck.co.uk/.

Local councils and health authorities collect information about the communities they serve. To see an example of what a statistical community profile might look like have a look at the examples from Swansea Council (Wales) https://www. swansea.gov.uk/communityareaprofiles?lang=en *and Cornwall (England)* https://www.cornwall.gov.uk/health-and-social-care/public-health/ joint-strategic-needs-assessment/community-and-health-based-profiles/. *An example from Alberta (Canada), aims to support older person service planning at* https://open.alberta.ca/publications/seniors-community-profile-olds.

Whilst data is important to help you identify community priorities, a health promoter will also need to do field research such as finding out about the history or culture of a community and the services, resources and assets in that area. Community profiles are situated in the present, so current issues such as climate change or the rising cost of living would also be included.

The concept of 'needs assessment' is similar to a community profile. They use similar data but a needs assessment is aimed at finding out what needs the community has. It does not usually look at the broader determinants or assets that a community has now and in the future.

COMMUNITY MOBILISATION

Community mobilisation is an approach where the community take action to collectively address an issue, and identify ways that they can act to change. Things that impact on whole communities need everyone to be part of the solution. This approach is often used where 'social norms' or attitudes need to be shifted for change to occur and where everyone in the community needs to be working together for action. It has been used commonly in areas like HIV and violence reduction where social norms or attitudes are major barriers to positive change. Resources with examples of community mobilisation for emergency preparedness, HIV and road safety are included at the end of the chapter.

COMMUNITY MOBILISATION AND ROAD SAFETY

SDG indicator 3.6 aims to halve the number of global deaths and injuries from road traffic accidents. In 2018, the WHO released a report highlighting road traffic injuries as the leading case of death in people aged 5–29 years (World Health Organization, 2018). Accompanying this report is an infographic that tells you how many people will die today, this year and this month from road traffic accidents https://extranet.who.int/roadsafety/death-on-the-roads/ as well as which countries have laws on seatbelts, drink driving, helmets and child seats. What is clear from this resource is how big the problem of road safety is across the world.

Health promotion in practice example: 20's plenty.

Community mobilisation has been used to advocate for a default 20 mph (30 kph) limit on roads. The organisation '20s Plenty for Us' at https:// www.20splenty.org/ is a non-profit organisation of over 600 local groups who are trying to campaign for a speed limit of 20 mph to be normal on residential roads in towns, villages and cities. Wales (UK) will be one of the first countries in the world to introduce laws to have a default 20 mph on roads where cars mix with cyclists and pedestrians. The ideas behind this are to reduce accidents, improve safety and also encourage more people to walk or cycle. You can read more at https://www.gov.wales/introducing-default-20mph-speed-limits.

COMMUNITY MOBILISATION TO REDUCE VIOLENCE AGAINST WOMEN AND GIRLS

SDG 16 is focussed on promoting peaceful and inclusive societies, which includes reducing all forms of violence. Community mobilisation is one of the strategies that has been used to reduce violence against women and girls. Gender-based violence includes the broad areas of physical, sexual, mental or other family violence against women and girls. Research suggests that gender-based violence is unacceptably high across the world. For example, intimate partner violence (IPV) prevalence by country suggests that on average 27% of ever-partnered women 15–49 years old have experienced physical or sexual violence at least once in their lifetime (Oram et al., 2022).

To reduce violence, we need to prevent it from happening in the first place. RESPECT women: Preventing violence against women (UN Women, 2020), is a framework with seven intervention areas. These are highlighted in Figure 3.8.

Figure 3.8 shows the intervention areas to reduce violence against women including a focus on relationship skills, women's empowerment, reducing poverty, providing services, making environments safe, preventing child and adolescent abuse and transforming attitudes, beliefs and social norms. Community mobilisation plays an important part in reducing violence through changing attitudes towards women and violence. You can see more on this resource including videos and examples from different country projects at https://www.unwomen.org/en/digital-library/publications/2020/07/respect-women-implementation-package.

The Oxfam Safe Families programme (Honda et al., 2022) in the Solomon Islands (A Pacific island nation) uses community mobilisation to transform harmful gender norms and end family violence. To do this, local attitudes to violence needed to be

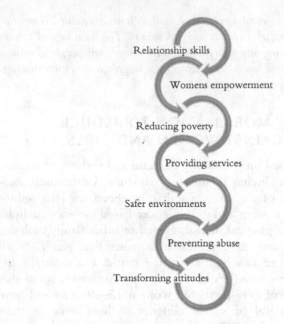

Figure 3.8 Intervention areas to reduce violence against women.

considered unacceptable, and to change this view four actions were needed:

(1) To mobilise communities to prevent and respond to violence.
(2) To promote collection action through coalitions.
(3) To build evidence and knowledge.
(4) To strengthen women's institutions, policies and laws.

Community mobilisation in this context recognises the role of not just individuals, but the structures, systems and services that can also support changes to gender norms. For example, to report violence there needs to be a reporting system, a justice system and a supportive health care system. Underpinning this needs to be laws and policies that protect women and their rights, for example, a 'bride price' (a custom where money is given by the groom to the bride's family), can undermine women's rights if women are seen as 'property'.

Health promotion in practice example: SASA! Uganda.

SASA! in Uganda is an evidence-based community mobilisation initiative that tackles social norms to prevent violence against women and girls. Their approach centres on addressing the male-dominated family structures which create norms where violence is acceptable. Resources include the SASA! activist kit and SASA! Faith for religious organisations. To see the SASA! story visit https://raisingvoices.org/women/sasa-approach/. SASA! has been used in different countries and UNAIDS, (2018) has created a resource about replicating the SASA! approach for HIV prevention. See wider reading at the end of the chapter.

COMMUNITY ACTION TO IMPROVE MEN'S HEALTH

On average men live fewer years than women and are more likely to die prematurely of suicide and male cancers such as prostate and testicular cancer. Community work with men has begun to focus on encouraging 'talking' in men to improve mental health, as well as reducing isolation and loneliness. Although in the UK rates of suicide are declining, they are higher in men especially young and mid-aged men who are less well-off and can show an increase during an economic downturn (Office of National Statistics, 2017). Research with mid-aged men suggests lack of purposeful activities, loss of employment, substance misuse and lack of significant support are all risk factors for suicide (The Samaritans, 2020). In response to this community action that focuses on building support, connections and job skills may hold promise for improving men's health.

'Movember' is an organisation which started with the idea of raising awareness of men's health by growing a 'Moustache (or 'Mo') in November – hence the name 'Movember'. One of the original ideas was that if you grew a 'Mo' people would ask you why you have one, and you could start a conversation about men's cancer, thereby increasing knowledge of men's health. This has since expanded into a much larger movement in different countries and includes a variety of issues that negatively impact the health of men including mental health, suicide and its prevention, and prostate and testicular cancer. See more at https://uk.movember.com/.

Health promotion in practice example: Making Connections Backpack (USA).
The 'Making Connections backpack toolkit' is a resource library for those
building community-level approaches to mental health and well-being with
men and boys. It has numerous practical resources to promote mental health
at the community level from just starting with an idea, to planning, im-
plementing, and delivering interventions at all levels of the community and
society. You can view the resource at https://preventioninstitute.org/
making-connections-backpack.

A large organisation which is growing in popularity is Men's
Sheds. Men's Sheds started in Australia as a space for men who
'don't talk face to face, they talk shoulder to shoulder' (Australian
Men's Shed Association, 2023). Men's sheds are community spaces
for men to do practical hobbies and activities across the UK. It is like
the idea of a garden or backyard shed where men would go to do
something practical by themselves. Most Men's Sheds' projects are
'bottom up' as they are run by the people who use them. Read
more about Australian Men's Sheds at https://mensshed.org/ and
UK Men's Sheds at www.menssheds.org.uk.

CHALLENGES OF COMMUNITY ACTION

Health is situated in the broader societal and political world. Challenges
such as the rising cost of living and climate change are national and
international challenges. Communities cannot solve everything, but
they can help to buffer the negative impacts of the problems they may
face. They can create real changes at the local level for local people.

The community engagement process is difficult to achieve, and the
process needs to be accessible to everyone. This will also be difficult if
people lack trust in others, do not know anything about each other, or
only perceive differences between themselves and others. There is a
section on 'Trust' in Chapter 2 'Developing personal skills', and a section
on inclusive healthcare in Chapter 5 'Reorientating healthcare services'.

Working in communities is not a short-term 'fix' and requires long-
term engagement. Groundwork UK (2019) highlights that one of the
biggest challenges facing communities taking action is securing
funding and having the skills to know where to go for support. Health
promoters are ideally placed to support communities in areas like this.

SUMMARY

Health promotion has its roots in community development where it works from the 'bottom' to support change, facilitate action and improve health and well-being. Recognising the strengths and assets that communities have, as well as ways to share power and decision making are essential to strong community action. The potential for communities to create action for change to improve health and tackle the social determinants of health is still underutilised and holds promise for the future of health promotion. The next chapter moves from communities to the wider environment and explores the 'settings' and places where we live, work and play.

WIDER READING

ONLINE

Audit Scotland (2019). Principles for community empowerment at https://www.audit-scotland.gov.uk/publications/principles-for-community-empowerment.

Buck, D., Wenzel, L., & Beech, J. (2021). Communities and health. The Kings Fund at https://www.kingsfund.org.uk/publications/communities-and-health.

Public Health England (2018). Guidance. Health matters: Community-centred approaches for health and well-being, https://www.gov.uk/government/publications/health-matters-health-and-wellbeing-community-centred-approaches/health-matters-community-centred-approaches-for-health-and-wellbeing.

Sendra, P., & Fitzpatrick, D. (2020). Community-led regeneration: A toolkit for residents and planners. UCL Press, available at https://www.uclpress.co.uk/products/125696#.

Think Local Act Personal (2023). A health and care transformation resource at https://www.thinklocalactpersonal.org.uk/.

World Health Organization (2020). Community engagement: A health promotion guide for universal health coverage in the hands of the people available at https://www.who.int/publications/i/item/9789240010529.

Community Mobilisation examples:

SBCC community mobilisation for action for emergency preparedness 'how to' guide at https://sbccimplementationkits.org/sbcc-in-emergencies/lessons/unit-3-community-mobilization/.

UNAIDS Communication mobilization for HIV with video examples at https://www.unaids.org/en/keywords/community-mobilization and UNAIDS (2018) replicating the SASA! approach at https://investment-book.unaids.org/sites/default/files/media_asset/Replicating_the_SASA_Approach.pdf.

TEXTBOOKS

Laverack, G. (2019). *Public health: Power, empowerment and professional practice.* Springer, London.

LISTENING AND WATCHING

TedX has some talks around community engagement such as:

'Bringing it home: lessons on community Engagement. Gretchen Krampf TEDxSanJuanIsland, https://www.youtube.com/watch?v=PQooUzvHEZc.

'Questions change everything in community engagement'. Max Hardy. TEDxStKilda Questions change everything in community engagement | Max Hardy | TEDxStKilda - YouTube.

'Sustainable community development: From what's wrong to what's strong'. Cormac Russell. TEDxExeter, https://www.youtube.com/watch?v=a5xR4QB1ADw.

ADDITIONAL REFERENCES

These are the additional references this chapter has used where electronic links have not been provided in the chapter.

Australian Men's Shed Association. (2023). Men don't talk face to face, they talk shoulder to shoulder. Available at https://mensshed.org/.

Aylward, B. L., Milford, K. M., Storey, K. E., Nykiforuk, C. I. J., & Raine, K. D. (2022). Local environment action on food project: Impact of a community-based food environment intervention in Canada. *Health Promotion International, 37*(2). 10.1093/heapro/daab127.

Buck, D., Wenzel, L., & Beech, J. (2021). Communities and health. Available at https://www.kingsfund.org.uk/publications/communities-and-health.

Cloete, E., & Dasig Salazar, A. (2022). "To be one with others": Exploring the development of community leadership in the Rural Philippines. *Development in Practice, 32*(6), 826–839. 10.1080/09614524.2022.2065244.

Communities Housing Trust. (2022). Case studies. Available at https://www.chtrust.co.uk/case-studies1.html.

Community Land Trust Network. (2022). What is a Community Land Trust CLT. Available at https://www.communitylandtrusts.org.uk/about-clts/what-is-a-community-land-trust-clt/.

Community Led Housing London. (2022). Community led housing projects in London. Available at https://www.communityledhousing.london/projects/.

Corbin, J. H., Oyene, U. E., Manoncourt, E., Onya, H., Kwamboka, M., Amuyunzu-Nyamongo, M., Sørensen, K., Mweemba, O., Barry, M. M., Munodawafa, D., Bayugo, Y. V., Huda, Q., Moran, T., Omoleke, S. A., Spencer-Walters, D., & Van den Broucke, S. (2021). A health promotion approach to emergency management: Effective community engagement strategies from five cases. *Health Promot Internat*, *36*(Supplement 1), i24–i38. 10.1093/heapro/daab152.

Department for Levelling Up. (2019). English indices of deprivation 2019: Mapping resources. Available at https://www.gov.uk/guidance/english-indices-of-deprivation-2019-mapping-resources#indices-of-deprivation-2019-explorer-postcode-mapper.

Douglas, H., Georgiou, A., & Westbrook, J. (2017). Social participation as an indicator of successful aging: an overview of concepts and their associations with health. *Aust Health Rev*, *41*(4), 455–462. 10.1071/ah16038.

Goodman, R. A., Bunnell, R., & Posner, S. F. (2014). What is "community health"? Examining the meaning of an evolving field in public health. *Prev Med*, *67*(Suppl 1), S58–S61. 10.1016/j.ypmed.2014.07.028.

Groundwork UK. (2019). Communities taking action. Undersanding the landscape for community action in the UK. Available at https://www.groundwork.org.uk/about-groundwork/reports/communities-taking-action/.

Honda, T., Homan, S., Leung, L., Bennett, A., Fulu, E., & Fisher, J. (2022). Community mobilisation in the framework of supportive social environment to prevent family violence in Solomon Islands. *World Development*, *152*, 105799. 10.1016/j.worlddev.2021.105799.

International Fund for Agricultural Development. (2023). Community gardens pave the way for climate-resilient agriculture in Gambia. Available at https://www.ifad.org/en.

Joshi, N., & Wende, W. (2022). Physically apart but socially connected: Lessons in social resilience from community gardening during the COVID-19 pandemic. *Landscape and Urban Planning*, *223*, 104418. 10.1016/j.landurbplan.2022.104418.

Kearns, A., & Whitley, E. (2020). Are housing and neighbourhood empowerment beneficial for mental health and wellbeing? Evidence from disadvantaged communities experiencing regeneration. *SSM Popul Health*, *12*, 100645. 10.1016/j.ssmph.2020.100645.

Lefkowich, M., Richardson, N., & Robertson, S. (2017). "If we want to get men in, then we need to ask men what they want": Pathways to Effective health programing for men. *American Journal of Mens Health*, *11*(5), 1512–1524. 10.1177/1557988315617825.

Marks, L., Laird, Y., Trevena, H., Smith, B. J., & Rowbotham, S. (2022). A scoping review of citizen science approaches in chronic disease prevention. *Front Public Health*, *10*, 743348. 10.3389/fpubh.2022.743348.

McGregor-Paterson, N. (2021). Learning from the community response to COVID-19; how the NHS can support communities to keep people well. Available at https://thehealthcreationalliance.org/wp-content/uploads/2021/04/THCA-Report_Community-response-to-COVID-19_NHS-learning-FINAL_-April-2021.pdf.

MIND. (2022). Peer support. Available at https://www.mind.org.uk/information-support/drugs-and-treatments/peer-support/about-peer-support/.

Morse, H., & Brown, A. (2021). Accessing local support online: Mothers' experiences of local Breastfeeding Support Facebook groups. *Maternal & Child Nutrition*, *17*(4), e13227. 10.1111/mcn.13227.

National Institute of Clinical Excellence. (2014). Maternal and child nutrition. Public health guideline [PH11]. Available at https://www.nice.org.uk/guidance/PH11/chapter/4-Recommendations#breastfeeding-3.

National Institute of Clinical Excellence. (2017). Community engagement: Improving health and wellbeing. Available at https://www.nice.org.uk/guidance/ng44/chapter/recommendations.

Nel, H. (2018). Community leadership: A comparison between asset-based community-led development (ABCD) and the traditional needs-based approach. *Development Southern Africa*, *35*(6), 839–851. 10.1080/0376835X.2018.1502075.

NHS England. (2017). Community capacity and peer support. Summary guide. Available at https://www.england.nhs.uk/wp-content/uploads/2017/06/516_Community-capacity-and-peer-support_S7.pdf.

Northern Ireland Statistics Research Agency. (2017). Northern Ireland multiple deprivation measure 2017. Available at https://www.nisra.gov.uk/statistics/deprivation/northern-ireland-multiple-deprivation-measure-2017-nimdm2017.

Office for Health Improvement and Disparities. (2022). Community centred practice: Applying all our health. Available at https://www.gov.uk/government/publications/community-centred-practice-applying-all-our-health.

Office of National Statistics. (2017). Who is at most risk of suicide? Available at https://www.ons.gov.uk/peoplepopulationandcommunity/birthsdeathsandmarriages/deaths/articles/whoismostatriskofsuicide/2017-09-07.

Oram, S., Fisher, H. L., Minnis, H., Seedat, S., Walby, S., Hegarty, K., Rouf, K., Angénieux, C., Callard, F., Chandra, P. S., Fazel, S., Garcia-Moreno, C., Henderson, M., Howarth, E., MacMillan, H. L., Murray, L. K., Othman, S., Robotham, D., Rondon, M. B., … Howard, L. M. (2022). The Lancet Psychiatry Commission on intimate partner violence and mental health: Advancing mental health services, research, and policy. *The Lancet Psychiatry*, *9*(6), 487–524. 10.1016/S2215-0366(22)00008-6.

Peters, L. E. R., Shannon, G., Kelman, I., & Meriläinen, E. (2022). Toward resourcefulness: Pathways for community positive health. *Global Health Promotion*, *29*(3), 5–13. 10.1177/17579759211051370.

Popay, J., Whitehead, M., Ponsford, R., Egan, M., & Mead, R. (2021). Power, control, communities and health inequalities I: Theories, concepts and analytical frameworks. *Health Promotion International*, *36*(5), 1253–1263. 10.1093/heapro/daaa133.

Public Health England. (2018). Health matters: Community-centred approaches for health and welleeing. Available at https://www.gov.uk/government/publications/health-matters-health-and-wellbeing-community-centred-approaches/health-matters-community-centred-approaches-for-health-and-wellbeing.

Scottish Government. Scottish Index of Multiple Deprivation 2020. Available at https://statistics.gov.scot/data/scottish-index-of-multiple-deprivation.

Shakya, P., Kunieda, M. K., Koyama, M., Rai, S. S., Miyaguchi, M., Dhakal, S., Sandy, S., Sunguya, B. F., & Jimba, M. (2017). Effectiveness of community-based peer support for mothers to improve their breastfeeding practices: A systematic review and meta-analysis. *PLoS One*, *12*(5), e0177434. 10.1371/journal.pone.0177434.

Slum soccer. (2023). Welcome to slum soccer. Available at https://slumsoccer.org/.

Social care institute for excellence. (2022). Co-production: What it is and how to do it. Available at https://www.scie.org.uk/co-production/what-how.

Sriram, V., Topp, S. M., Schaaf, M., Mishra, A., Flores, W., Rajasulochana, S. R., & Scott, K. (2018). 10 best resources on power in health policy and systems in low- and middle-income countries. *Health Policy Plan*, *33*(4), 611–621. 10.1093/heapol/czy008.

The Samaritans. (2020). Out of sight, out of mind. Available at https://media.samaritans.org/documents/Samaritans_-_out_of_sight_out_of_mind_2020.pdf.

Think Local Act Personal. (2021). Ladder of co-production. Available at https://www.thinklocalactpersonal.org.uk/Browse/Co-production/.

Truong, S., Gray, T., & Ward, K. (2022). Enhancing urban nature and place-making in social housing through community gardening. *Urban Forestry & Urban Greening*, *72*, 127586. 10.1016/j.ufug.2022.127586.

UK Centre for Ecology and Hydrology. (2022). *Citizen science resources.* Available at https://www.ceh.ac.uk/citizen-science.

UN Women. (2020). RESPECT Women: Preventing violence against women – Implementation package. Available at https://www.unwomen.org/en/digital-library/publications/2020/07/respect-women-implementation-package.

UNAIDS. (2018). Replicating the SASA! approach. Available at at https://investment-book.unaids.org/sites/default/files/media_asset/Replicating_the_SASA_Approach.pdf.

Welsh Government. (2019). Welsh Index of Multiple Deprivation. https://statswales.gov.wales/Catalogue/Community-Safety-and-Social-Inclusion/Welsh-Index-of-Multiple-Deprivation.

Wigan Council. (2018). Small things make a great deal – Wigan Council. Available at https://www.youtube.com/watch?v=ef0lF6qmBt0.

World Health Organization. (1978). Declaration of Alma Ata. Available at https://cdn.who.int/media/docs/default-source/documents/almaata-declaration-en.pdf?sfvrsn=7b3c2167_2.

World Health Organization. (2018). Global status report on road safety 2018. Available at https://www.who.int/publications/i/item/9789241565684.

World Health Organization. (2022). Universal Health Coverage. Available at https://www.who.int/news-room/fact-sheets/detail/universal-health-coverage-(uhc).

4

CREATING SUPPORTIVE
ENVIRONMENTS

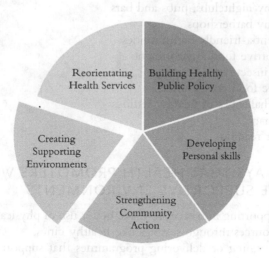

Figure 4.1 Creating supportive environments.

DOI: 10.4324/9781003462323-5

- Five ways that health promoters work to create supportive environments
- Overview
- Healthy settings
- Healthy cities
- Sustainable water and 'dry cities'
- Healthy islands
- Health promoting schools
- Healthy universities
- Healthy prisons
- Faith-based settings
- Health at work
- Eliminating workplace violence
- Mental well-being at work
- The five ways to well-being at work
- Alternative settings for health promotion
- Healthy nightclubs, pubs and bars
- Healthy barbershops
- Dementia-friendly communities
- Supportive food environments
- Food insecurity
- Online food environments
- The challenges of healthy settings
- Summary
- Wider reading

FIVE WAYS THAT HEALTH PROMOTERS WORK TO CREATE SUPPORTIVE ENVIRONMENTS

(1) Supporting initiatives to make better use of physical or natural resources through settings like healthy cities.

(2) Designing or delivering programmes that support the health and well-being of those using settings like a workplace.

(3) Working with organisations to achieve specific standards such as healthy schools.

(4) Delivering health promotion interventions through traditional (school) and non-traditional (barbers) settings.

(5) Working with organisations to modify existing spaces to be inclusive, safe and accessible for all (Figure 4.1).

OVERVIEW

A healthy environment supports health and well-being and is safe and accessible for everyone. A well-designed environment encourages good health. Think about where you live. How easy is it for you to get to your nearest green space like a park or wood, or a blue space like a beach or lake? Maybe you just have to walk for five minutes? Perhaps you have to drive or take a bus? Think about this green or blue space. Is it safe? Is it free? Is it accessible to everyone? Is it free of litter or pollution? Does it have public toilets? Are there rules about what you can do here? Are there risks from nature such as erosion or flooding? These factors impact our ability to use green and blue spaces and consequently can impact our health. These factors can be grouped under four domains; the natural environment, the built environment, the social-cultural environment, and the policy environment. These are shown in Figure 4.2.

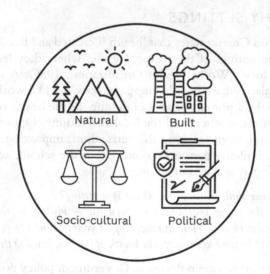

Figure 4.2 Supportive environment domains.

Figure 4.2 shows four supportive environment domains.

- The natural environment includes ecosystems, climate, geography and nature.
- The built environment includes buildings, infrastructures like transport systems and pollution.
- The social-cultural environment includes safe, accessible, equal and inclusive social and cultural spaces.
- The policy environment includes laws, good governance and political stability.

The four domains can affect health in different ways but a supportive environment needs to include all four areas. Take the example of people who work on a construction site; protection from the weather (the natural environment), using non-toxic building materials (built environment), following norms such as wearing hard hats (social-cultural environment), and health and safety law (policy environment) are all integral to creating a safe construction site. We will use these four domains more later in this chapter.

HEALTHY SETTINGS

The Ottawa Charter states that 'health is created and lived by people within the settings of their everyday life; where they learn, work, play and love' (World Health Organization, 1986). A setting is a space or place where people engage in activities like work or study. For example, a primary school can influence the health of children, parents/carers, teachers and the local community. Opportunities to do this come from teaching the curriculum, improving the school buildings, building partnerships outside of the school, active travel plans, safe play spaces and so on.

Practitioner skills activity 4a: What is a setting?
List all the places that you have been in, or visited, in the last week (indoors and outdoors). How did they impact your health? Do you think any of these could be used to promote the health of the people using those settings?

Healthy settings are reflected in Government policy documents in many countries including 'healthy hospitals', 'healthy schools', 'healthy cities' and 'healthy workplaces'. Healthy settings focus on the wider determinants of health and acknowledge that these determinants interact with people in that setting. For example, how people travel to work impacts health. Workplaces might focus on promoting active travel to work to improve employee health. This might involve reviewing the ways people can reach the workplace through public transport routes or better road design, supporting people with buying equipment like bicycles or providing facilities to those who actively travel to work like bike storage.

The original healthy settings approaches were based on participatory health promotion which suggested that everyone within a setting had a shared responsibility to change. Peterson et al. (2002) created a framework showing the areas that are important to a healthy setting. The seven areas are:

- Partnerships.
- Positive health values.
- Availability of services.
- Access to facilities/resources.
- Community focussed.
- Health behaviour change support.
- Social systems support.

Partnerships are important for creating health within organisations such as partnering with catering companies or service providers. **Organisations** with positive health values are more likely to prioritise the health of those using those settings. **Availability and access** to facilities and services like gym membership support behaviour change. **Community focussed** means interventions should be appropriate and tailored to the people using those settings. **Behaviour change support** and **social systems support** refer to networks, peers or other support that facilitates change.

Examples of how these seven areas are relevant to settings can be seen in the health promotion in practice example below on menstrual equity and period poverty.

Health promotion in practice example: Period poverty and menstrual equity.
All women should be able to manage their periods safely and with dignity.

Being unable to do so has a major impact on emotional and physical well-being. An example of 'available services' and 'access to facilities and resources' is the provision of period-friendly toilets that are accessible and safe. This means toilets with a door and lock, soap and washing facilities and appropriate waste disposable. For more on menstrual equity see https://www.freedom4girls.co.uk/.

Period poverty refers to the inability to purchase and access period products during a menstrual cycle. An example of 'partnerships' and 'available services' is the UK Department for Education (Department for Education, 2022) free period product scheme for schools and colleges. An example of 'community focussed' are organisations that are working to provide period products to vulnerable groups such as homeless women or those living in refugee camps see https://periodpoverty.uk/.

Healthy settings have since evolved from a convenient location to deliver health promotion to incorporate broader health promotion actions such as creating healthy public policy. See Chapter 6 'Healthy public policy' for more examples. The Sustainable Development Goals (SDGs) outlined in chapter 1 include healthy settings, for example, healthy cities. The 'healthy dry cities' example below shows this move away from a setting being a convenient location to a setting incorporating policy and governance in creating supportive environments.

HEALTHY CITIES

SDG 11 aspires to 'make cities and human settlements inclusive, safe, resilient and sustainable' (United Nations, 2015). This includes giving access to affordable housing, sustainable transport, and safe inclusive green spaces. As more people live in cities than in rural areas the inclusion of the 'city' in the SDGs seems logical. But how can we achieve a healthy city? Cities are often industrial, busy, commercial hives of activity that keep evolving and growing. The WHO 'European Healthy Cities' concept is centred on what a city is, and what a city could become in the future. The main goals of 'Healthy Cities' includes advocating for equity in policy, creating supportive environments that can support the health and well-being of residents, promoting healthy urban planning and supporting communities with health action. The WHO's 'European Healthy Cities Network' outlines six core themes in health cities. These are highlighted in Figure 4.3.

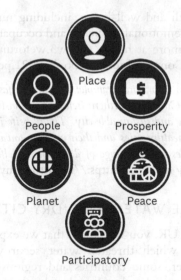

Figure 4.3 shows that healthy cities aspire to be a place of community prosperity, that they are participatory, and activities are done to obtain health and peace. Healthy cities lead by example, they look after their populations so people can fulfil their full potential. To achieve this, health has to be on the policy agenda of cities and in their planning and development for the future.

Practitioner skills activity 4b: What makes a healthy city?
Think about a city that you have visited. If you have not visited a city, you could try taking a virtual tour of a city using a website. Using the six themes of a healthy city, if you were going to improve the city give examples of what you could do in each of the six areas. You could look at how to increase prosperity, how to encourage community engagement or how to support the creation of safe, clean or green environments.

The World Economic Forum (2021) provides a guide for private and public organisations in developing effective partnerships that promote healthy living in cities. They suggest different examples from over 100 cities and eight areas where partnerships could work to promote health and well-being, including nutrition, sanitation, physical activity, emotional resilience and occupational and financial well-being. See more at https://www3.weforum.org/docs/WEE_ Healthy_Cities_Communities_Playbook_2021.pdf.

Health promotion in practice example: Healthy Belfast (Northern Ireland).
Belfast Healthy Cities in Northern Ireland has a vision to be recognised as a healthy, equitable and sustainable city. The website includes a wide range of resources about healthy cities and their progress towards their vision. The website also includes a wide range of data about Belfast based on the six themes of a healthy city. Visit https://belfasthealthycities.com/.

SUSTAINABLE WATER AND 'DRY CITIES'

If you live in the UK, you will know that we experience temporary water shortages which threaten water security in the summer months. However, some countries and regions experience water shortages all year round as they have low levels of fresh water and/or rain. SDG 6 is to 'ensure availability and sustainable management of water and sanitation for all'. This includes a focus on improving water quality, increasing water use efficiency, reducing pollution, and increasing safe reuse practices. Some cities struggle to provide fresh water to the people that live there, and this requires urgent action.

Practitioner skills activity 4c: Safe water.
Approximately 74% of the population are using safely managed drinking water services globally (World Health Organization, 2022). About 45% of household wastewater generated globally is discharged with no safe treatment. Why do you think some people lack access to a safely managed drinking water source? Why is so much household water not safely treated?

Dry cities are mostly situated in arid places, with low levels of fresh water and/or rain. Many are located in the Middle East (i.e. Iran), or North Africa (i.e. Libya) and some are 'desert cities' like Las Vegas (USA). Cities can also be temporarily dry through drought or inadequate infrastructures for water supply, management,

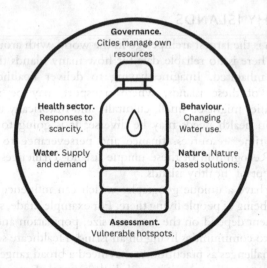

Figure 4.4 Six policy areas for dry cities.

distribution or storage. The British Medical Journal (BMJ) has resources on dry cities including videos and infographics which you can see at https://www.bmj.com/healthy-dry-cities. They suggest six policy areas for dry cities to work on which are shown in Figure 4.4.

The six policy areas that help to create change in dry cities include:

• Health sector planning for more frequent problems such as heat-related illness.
• Good governance practices such as giving cities autonomy to manage their resources.
• Water and water management improvement in supply and demand.
• Behaviour change including behaviours people need to manage extreme heat or conserve water.
• Nature-based solutions such as planting trees for shade.

HEALTHY ISLANDS

Indonesia is the largest archipelago in the world, with around 17,000 islands. There is no reliable data for how many islands there are or that are inhabited. Imagine having to deliver healthcare across hundreds of these islands, where transport may be infrequent, communities might be small, culturally and historically unique and population health needs may be diverse. It is going to take considerable time, resources, finance and perseverance to reach everyone. Recognition of these unique 'island' challenges has led to the concept of 'healthy islands'.

Islands have a unique geography which can influence the health and well-being of people living there. For example, trade, services and employment depend on the location, size, population and resources available to communities living on an island. Healthcare services face unique challenges as practitioners may need a broad range of skills to work in remote communities with little support. Even standard interventions that rely on information technology can be problematic with limited internet services or poor mobile phone coverage.

The Pacific island countries (for example, Fiji and Samoa) were the first to use the concept of 'healthy islands'. A meeting in 1995 created the Yanuca Island Declaration on Health (World Health Organization, 2015). It says that healthy islands should be five things: places where children are nurtured, environments that invite learning and leisure, a place where people work and age with dignity, where ecological balance is a source of pride, and the ocean that sustains us is protected. These are shown in Figure 4.5 'Healthy islands'.

The declaration echoes the original ideas of healthy settings and SDGs like 14 'life below water' that highlights the importance of conserving coastal areas and marine habitats. Challenges like rising sea levels through climate change, overfishing or pollution threaten many island communities and looking after resources like the ocean are vital to support communities and sustain livelihoods.

Practitioner skills activity 4d: Creating sustainable island solutions.

SDG 8 'decent work and economic growth' includes devising and implementing policies to promote sustainable tourism that creates jobs and promotes local culture and products. Imagine you are working with a group of island communities like the Isles of Scilly (England) that has around 2,000

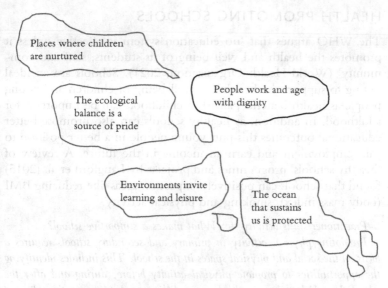

Figure 4.5 Healthy islands.

*residents. The main island has a primary school, a health centre and one
street with shops, cafes and hotels. Tourism to the island is an important
source of revenue and many people come to the islands for holidays, but their
visits create a lot of waste that cannot be recycled. What could you do to
promote sustainable tourism and create jobs or promote local products at the
same time? Can you connect your ideas to Figure 4.5?*

Health promotion in practice example: Healthy islands in Scotland.

*Scotland has the most islands in the UK nations. The Healthy Islands
Fund in Scotland has been created by the Scottish Government to improve
the quality of life of people living on the 93 inhabited islands in Scotland.
The National Plan for Scotland's Islands (Scottish Government, 2019) has
13 objectives to improve the quality of life in the islands through four approaches; fair, integrated, green and inclusive. Although objective 7 is ex-
plicitly focussed on 'improving health, social care and well-being', many
others have a significant influence on health, such as improving housing and
transport services. You can read more about the projects and the Islands Fund
at* https://www.inspiringscotland.org.uk/.

HEALTH PROMOTING SCHOOLS

The WHO argues that 'no education system is effective unless it promotes the health and well-being of its students, staff and community' (World Health Organization, 2021). Schools are an ideal setting to support the health and well-being of children and young people as health benefits gained in childhood can be important for adulthood. In addition, as healthy schools can also promote better educational outcomes this puts young people in a better position to gain employment and earn an income in the future. A review of 'healthy schools' programmes and projects by Langford et al. (2015) found that schools can positively impact on areas like reducing BMI (body mass index), smoking and physical activity.

Practitioner skills activity 4e: What makes a supportive school?

Promoting physical activity in primary and secondary schools requires a focus on the social and physical spaces in the school. This includes identifying the opportunities to promote physical activity before, during and after the school day. What do you think is needed to create a supportive physical activity environment in a primary or secondary school? Who could be involved in promoting physical activity before, during and after school?

SDG 4 focuses on 'ensuring inclusive and equitable quality education', with targets around the building and upgrading the education of facilities that are child, disability and gender sensitive, as well as safe and inclusive learning environments. The World Health Organization (2021) has guidance on how to make every school a health promotion school. It suggests eight global standards for a health-promoting school system. Figure 4.6 shows these:

The first three standards (Government commitment and investment, school and community investment, school governance and leadership support) focus on leadership and governance which are needed to ensure that health is considered a priority in everything the school does.

The other five standards are closely focused on the school itself. These include:

- Partnerships with local communities. These can involve parents or carers of children or local organisations like faith communities.
- The curriculum. This includes physical, social and emotional

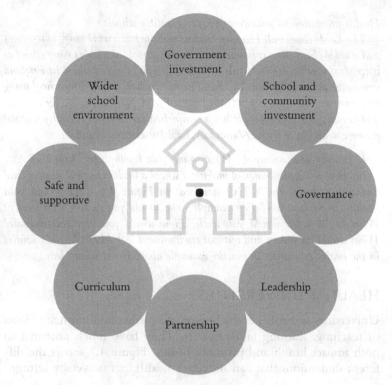

Figure 4.6 Standards of a health promoting school.

health. In the UK, PSHE (personal, social, health and economic) education is a legal requirement. It teaches relationships and sex education, mental health, personal safety, digital literacy and money. You can read more about this at the PSHE Association website https://pshe-association.org.uk/.

- A safe and supportive school. This is about making sure when children come to school they are safe from harm and their mental and emotional well-being is looked after.
- The wider school physical environment. This is indoor spaces such as buildings that are free from hazards, and outdoor spaces like safe spaces to play.
- School-based health services. These include services that meet the needs of young people like the provision of a school nursing service or child and adolescent mental health services.

Health promotion in practice example: Healthy schools.

The Leeds (England) Healthy Schools website has a wide range of resources and a video about what is important in health schools available to any school at https://www.healthyschools.org.uk/. If you attended school in England you can search to see if your childhood primary school is a healthy school using this link. In Northern Ireland, the Anna Freud National centre for children and families and young people has a comprehensive 'mentally healthy schools' resource available at https://mentallyhealthyschools.org.uk/.

Practitioner skills activity 4f: What would your healthy school look like?

Imagine you are in charge of making a school a healthier school in your local community. Using the WHO standards in Figure 4.6, what would your healthy school look like? For example, who would you partner with locally? What health topics would you teach? How would you keep children safe? What would the indoor and outdoor environment look like? Use the resources in the health promotion in practice example above if you want ideas.

HEALTHY UNIVERSITIES

Universities and colleges for higher and further education are places of teaching, learning and research. They have much potential to both impact health and promote health. Figure 4.7 shows the different dimensions that can influence health in a university setting.

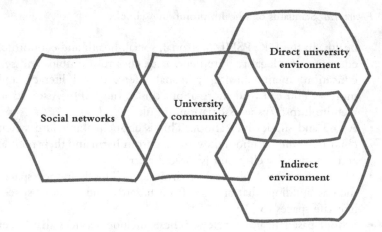

Figure 4.7 Healthy university dimensions.

Figure 4.7 shows the dimensions that can impact those working or studying in universities. At the centre are students and staff who make up the university community. The second dimension is social networks. This includes friends, colleagues, peers and the learning, teaching and research activities that take place. It also includes social opportunities such as clubs and societies. The third dimension has two parts. The university environment influences people directly and indirectly. Direct-level environments include the structures and policies that influence the university's environment, such as student and staff policies, academic, health and leisure facilities and the physical environment such as indoor and outdoor spaces. Indirect-level environments are outside the direct control of the university such as immigration or employment rules, where the university is situated, accommodation and transportation options, future employment opportunities and healthcare systems.

The Okanagan Charter (International Conference on Health Promoting Universities and Colleges, 2015) is an international charter for health-promoting universities and colleges. The charter encourages universities and colleges to create healthy campuses outlining how they can 'transform the health and sustainability of our current and future societies, strengthen communities and contribute to the well-being of people, places and the planet' (p. 2).

The Okanagan Charter has two calls to action; to embed health into the culture of universities across all levels, and to lead health promotion action locally and globally. The principles underpinning the Okanagan Charter are similar to the Ottawa Charter for Health Promotion (World Health Organization, 1986), and include action on reorientating health services, and creating campus policies and supportive environments for health. You can read more about the charter at the University of British Columbia (Canada) at https:// wellbeing.ubc.ca/okanagan-charter. Waterworth (2017) has practical advice on how the charter can be applied in New Zealand which explains each action area and how it can be used (see reference list at the end of the chapter).

Practitioner skills activity 4g: Healthy universities and student safety.

Imagine you were designing a health promotion campaign for improving student safety on a university or college campus in your local area. What sort of actions would you do for students and staff? What could the university do that would support campus safety for example by creating supportive campus environments? Use the resources in the health promotion in practice example below for ideas.

The concept of healthy universities focuses on creating a learning environment that promotes the health and well-being of those studying and working within universities and colleges. Healthy universities are not just about working with an individual but creating supportive environments. Universities UK (2023) has a wide variety of resources which help to illustrate this point. For example, The 'Stepchange' framework advocates for universities to prioritise mental health in their organisation and their policies, and the resource 'Spiking what universities can do', explores action measures to reduce drink spiking. Drink spiking is adding something to someone's drink, like a drug. There is also guidance for universities on suicide-safer universities. You can read more at https://www.universitiesuk.ac.uk/ what-we-do/policy-and-research/publications?topic=42.

Health promotion in practice example: Mentally healthy universities (UK).
The mental health charity MIND (2023) has trialled a mentally healthy university programme. The programme has five areas including equipping students with the knowledge to manage their mental health, reducing stigma, and supporting students to manage their mental health in future work. It also has training for staff mental health champions and staff mental health peer supporters to provide support and reduce stigma around mental health in universities. Read more at https://www.mind.org.uk/workplace/ mentally-healthy-universities-programme/.

Globally there is a wide range of resources to promote healthy universities. The UK Universities Network toolkit has a wide range of resources to support universities, including a self-review tool, case studies, resources and links to international healthy university networks. Read more at https://healthyuniversities.ac.uk/toolkit-and-resources/. The international sustainable campus network is a global network of information sharing to promote sustainability in universities with a wide range of examples from projects across the world. Read more at https:// international-sustainable-campus-network.org/. 'StudentMinds' in the UK https://www.studentminds.org.uk/ also provides a wide range of resources for students and universities to promote mental health and well-being.

Health promotion in practice example: Reducing sexual harassment and violence in universities.

Lewis (2022) in a UK Parliament research briefing suggests a significant number of students in post-18 studies experience sexual harassment and violence during their time in higher education. Female students are most likely to experience this, and male students are the most likely to perpetuate it. The Office for Students (2023) has collated a wide range of resources for student safety around sexual harassment hate crime and online harassment from UK universities. Read and see more at https://www.officeforstudents. org.uk/advice-and-guidance/student-wellbeing-and-protection/re-sources-for-student-safety-and-wellbeing/.

HEALTHY PRISONS

The global prison population exceeds 11 million people, and with this increased number comes overcrowded prison systems (World Prison Brief, 2023). There is over-reliance on criminal justice systems to deal with crime, rather than preventing crime through policies that promote social justice and reduce inequalities. People who enter the criminal justice system have poorer physical health and mental health than the general population. For example, in a report found in England and Wales that approximately 48% of men and 70% of women in prison experience mental health difficulties (Criminal Justice Joint Inspection, 2021). Poor mental health can be both a causal factor in crime and a consequence of engagement in the criminal justice system. Consequences of poor mental health include suicide which is the leading cause of death in prisons in nearly all European countries (World Health Organization, 2023). There is also an increasing number of older people in prisons who may have a range of chronic conditions which prisons are not well equipped to deal with.

Nelson Mandela said that *'no one truly knows a nation until one has been inside its jails. A nation should not be judged by how it treats its highest citizens, but by its lowest ones'* — cited on the UN website (2023). This quote is used in support of the 'United Nations Standard for the Minimum Rules of the Treatment of Prisoners' (United Nations Office on Drugs and Crime, 2015), also known as the 'Mandela Rules'. The rules are designed to improve prison conditions. These rules state that prisoners should be treated with respect, and protected from degrading treatment and punishment, their safety should be ensured, and they should be provided with nutritional food and access to daily exercise. Healthcare provision should be of the same standard of care as in the community. The World Health Organization supports this notion, as has a range of prison reports and examples across Europe at https://www.who.int/europe/health-topics/prisons-and-health.

There are major differences in the quality of prison systems across the world. Some countries like the UK have regular prison inspections and follow specific procedures to support and maintain the health and welfare of those in prisons. For example, skills based courses to help prisoners learn skills and education opportunities to improve education or literacy are provided. Many prisoners also get paid for their work in prisons (UK Government, 2023). In Scotland, the prison system is unique in that it has made an explicit commitment to health promotion (Woodall & Freeman, 2021). See the health promotion in practice example below for more on healthy prisons in Scotland.

Health promotion in practice example: Healthy prisons in Scotland (UK).

Scotland has a health promotion in prisons framework including 11 pillars of health promotion action (Brutus, 2012). These are tobacco, alcohol, illicit drugs, mental health, healthy eating, oral health, sexual relationships, the transmission of blood-borne viruses, physical activity, parenting and long-term conditions. These are achieved through the 'unifiers' of the prisoner involvement, supportive environments and policies, community and service involvement and evaluation. You can view the framework and other documents around healthy prisons at https://www.scotphn.net/projects/offender-health-2/offender-health/. An example of action can be found on the NHS Forth Valley website at https://nhsforthvalley.com/health-services/health-promotion/prisons/.

Across Europe, research from the prison health status report (World Health Organization, 2023) illustrates that supporting prisoners' health is doing well in some areas, such as Covid-19 vaccination rates and the provision of education and employment. However, there are large differences in screening and treatment for communicable diseases such as HIV across Europe. There is also variable availability of free products to protect people from risky behaviours such as needle exchanges, condoms or PrEP availability which is recommended for those at risk of HIV (National Institute for Clinical Excellence, 2022b).

Outside of Europe low- and middle-income countries appear to be doing less well in prison health. Many prisoners globally experience considerable hardship and a deprivation of human rights. A study in 39 sub-Saharan African countries exploring young people in prison (aged 12 to 18) found that prisons did not meet the basic needs of young people and violated human rights (Van Hout & Mhlanga-Gunda, 2019). The study highlights issues such as overcrowding, poor sanitation and hygiene, poor quality food, lack of access to healthcare and threats of violence and abuse. Other studies from sub-Saharan African countries also report similar findings. Diendéré et al. (2021) note in Burkina Faso that 'humanizing prisons' is essential, and areas such as hygiene, sanitation, overcrowding and food quality need to improve.

These examples show that more work is needed in many countries to improve prison conditions and to encourage the achievement of the 'Mandela Rules'. For more guidance on prison reform and alternatives to imprisonment, the United Nations Office on Drugs and Crime has an extensive collection of toolkits, publications and reports at https://www.unodc.org/unodc/en/justice-and-prison-reform/cpcj-prison-reform.html.

FAITH-BASED SETTINGS

In the UK there are high levels of self-reported religious identification in Black and Asian Minority Ethnic groups (BAME), and places of worship can bring BAME together for a common purpose (Tomalin et al., 2019). This suggests opportunities in places of worship to promote and support health. Work by Dunn et al. (2021) found that most interventions for physical activity and healthy eating in faith-based settings showed at least one behaviour change. The organisation Faith Action (2023) shows how the NHS and local authorities work with faith groups, as well as promoting the value of faith-based groups to reduce inequalities, for example through social prescribing and reducing loneliness and isolation. You can read more at https://www.faithaction.net/our-resources/.

Faith-based communities and organisations are often engaged with health and well-being concerns. For example, the Birmingham (England) faith community map, shows how more than 700 places of worship are supporting their communities. The map is designed to direct faith communities to support the areas that have the greatest need. You can view the map at https://footstepsbcf.org.uk/birmingham-faith-community-map/.

Health promotion in practice example: Faith-based partnerships.

Faith-based partnerships can work to improve health in communities with a strong faith connection. For example, the organisation 'Christians working in global health' work across six continents and advocate for equal access to quality healthcare. Their work includes partnership projects such as the five-year SCOPE project to prevent maternal and child mortality through community engagement in four countries. Read more at https://www.ccih.org/scope/. The organisation was also part of a faith-based partnership that created a family planning advocacy project in Kenya and Zambia. Churches were used to promote family planning advocacy and research by Bornet et al. (2021) shows the strategies they used. See the reference list at the end for the link.

One of the challenges with faith-based settings is the lack of evidence-supporting interventions. Difficulties include a lack of published best practices and intervention outcomes are likely to be different depending on the place of worship contexts such as faith, location, leaders and congregations. Most evidence comes from African American church-based programmes in the USA which historically has some well-known interventions. 'Body & Soul' and 'Healthy body, health spirit' which are both aimed at promoting a healthy diet are two such examples. You can read about both interventions and view their resources including cookbooks, videos, handouts, posters, interventions, and a gospel walking tape at Body & Soul https://ebccp.cancercontrol.cancer.gov/programDetails.do?programId=257161 or Healthy body, healthy spirit https://ebccp.cancercontrol.cancer.gov/programDetails.do?programId=220755.

Health promotion in practice example: Mosques and health.

'Healthy living in mosques' (Public Health England, 2017) is a resource to support mosques in their health promotion work. It provides mosque leaders and communities with evidence of best practices and shows how health promotion can be linked to Islamic teachings. Read more at https://www.

gov.uk/government/publications/healthy-living-mosques. *It also highlights examples such as 'Talking from the heart' to support mental and emotional health with short films available in Somali, Urdu and Bengali. See more at* http://www.talkingfromtheheart.org/.

HEALTH AT WORK

The workplace is an important setting for health promotion. Many adults spend a lot of their time at work and this presents opportunities for health promotion. Experiences of work vary and impact people differently. For example, some workplaces have workplace hazards that can impact on health. This might be long shift work such as in a factory or exposure to harmful substances such as manufacturing work. Some workers may also experience more vulnerabilities in a workplace such as lone workers or may have fewer rights than others such as casual, temporary or migrant workers.

Practitioner skills activity 4h: Covid-19 and workplace health.

During the Covid-19 pandemic, some countries were 'locked-down' meaning there were restrictions on what people could do. Some people could not work as non-essential businesses were closed, and others were expected to work remotely or continued their work as normal. Identify the different ways that the Covid-19 lockdown may have impacted the experiences of these different groups of workers; teachers, hospital managers, gym instructors, and builders. What did employers do in your country (if anything) for workers or workplaces?

SDG target 8.5 says there should be 'equal pay for work of equal value'. But, there are still differences in what people get paid for the work they do. Income is a major determinant of health (The Health Foundation, 2022). Some jobs pay more than others depending on the type of job and jobs that require more skills or responsibility are usually paid more. However, there are also differences in pay in the same jobs. The gender pay gap in the UK shows that on average, men are paid more than women. This means that women are taking home less money than men. Women are also much less likely to progress into high-paying senior roles and high-paying sectors are made up of more male workers. This can impact negatively the health of women. You can look up UK companies and see what the pay gap is at https://gender-pay-gap.service.gov.uk/. In the UK, there is also a disability pay gap and an ethnicity pay gap.

Workplace healthy lifestyle interventions have been found to improve health and well-being (Sidossis et al., 2021). Employers can support their workforce in many different ways. Three different examples are presented below; eliminating workplace violence, mental well-being at work, and the five ways to well-being.

ELIMINATING WORKPLACE VIOLENCE

Some areas of health and well-being in a workplace can only be addressed through organisational change. Reducing or eliminating workplace violence, bullying, harassment, discrimination or accidents cannot be reduced without considering the workplace setting. There is an individual component to these areas, for example, offering violence training de-escalation or health and safety training. However, the places in which these hazards or risks occur require more than a well-trained workforce.

Wirth et al. (2021) looked at interventions to reduce violence in Emergency Departments (EDs) where people attend emergency care. EDs have multiple risk factors for violence including high-stress spaces and overcrowding. They suggest that stressors in the environment that lead to violence and how organisations respond to these are important in the prevention of violence. Figure 4.2 shows four different environment domains. They can be applied to this example to show how violence occurs through different environmental conditions. If there are no adequate risk assessments in place (policy environment), limited support for staff who experience violence (social-cultural environment), the space is crowded and uncomfortable (built environment), or those waiting are too hot or too cold (natural environment), then workplace violence risks remain. Tackling workplace violence in the context of EDs requires multicomponent interventions, meaning they include individuals, the organisation, and the different elements of the environment.

Practitioner skills activity 4i: Healthy transport hubs.

Think of a busy transport hub like a train or bus station or an air or sea port near you. Identify the different types of jobs that people might do in these spaces. Using Figure 4.2 to help you, what domains of the environment might impact on the health and safety of people working in the station or port? Are some workers more vulnerable than others? If you wanted to improve the health of those working in these spaces what would you suggest at the four different environment domains in Figure 4.2?

MENTAL WELL-BEING AT WORK

NICE guidance on mental well-being at work suggests a three-tiered approach to improving mental well-being in the workplace (National Institute for Clinical Excellence, 2022a). This is illustrated in Figure 4.8. The bottom tier is 'organisation', the middle tier is 'individual' and the top tier is 'targeted'.

The bottom tier is organisation. To improve mental health in a workplace an organisation could seek to use accreditation or charters to improve employee health through a workplace well-being charter. Managers could be trained in Mental Health First Aid to support their employees. Organisations could also provide access to resources to services that support health, such as suitable office furniture and physical activity or recreational opportunities. For an example of a 'Well-being at Work' charter see https://healthatworkcentre.org.uk/

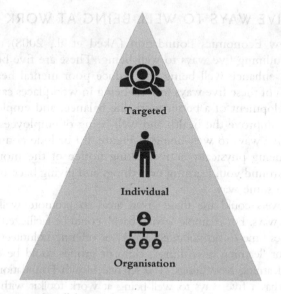

Figure 4.8 Mental well-being three-tiered approach.

wellbeing-charter/ and for Mental Health First Aid resources see https://www.mentalhealthatwork.org.uk/organisation/mental-health-first-aid-england/.

The middle tier is 'individual'. To improve employee mental health, employees could be given opportunities to talk about mental health, offered activities around the five ways to well-being (see the five ways to well-being section below) or encouraged to complete an employee wellness action plan. An example of a wellness action plan from MIND is at this link https://www.mind.org.uk/workplace/mental-health-at-work/taking-care-of-yourself/.

The top tier is 'targeted'. This uses similar interventions to the middle tier but focusses on employees who are at risk of poor mental health such as those who are more vulnerable in some way, for example, they work in a high-risk occupation. Those working in emergency services may work in particularly high-risk jobs. Organisations like 'Blue Light Together' is a charity that supports UK emergency services staff to look after their mental health. https://bluelighttogether.org.uk/.

THE FIVE WAYS TO WELL-BEING AT WORK

The New Economics Foundation (Aked et al., 2008) released a report outlining five ways to well-being. These are five behaviours that can enhance well-being and reduce poor mental health. The inclusion of these five ways to well-being in workplaces can support the development of a better work-life balance, and employer support can improve the health and well-being of employees.

The five ways to well-being in Figure 4.9 include connecting to others, being physically active, taking notice of the moment and what is around you, learning new things and giving back by helping others in some way.

Employers could use these given areas to promote well-being in different ways. For example 'giving back', could be facilitated by giving employees time to do volunteer work, or offering volunteer opportunities. For 'learning new things', clubs or groups could be created to support learning new things. The Mental Health Foundation in New Zealand has a five ways to well-being at work toolkit with activities, games and resources at https://mentalhealth.org.nz/resources/resource/

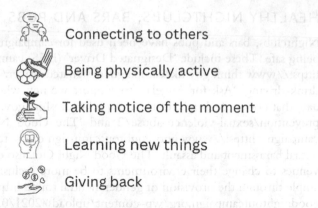

Connecting to others

Being physically active

Taking notice of the moment

Learning new things

Giving back

Figure 4.9 The five ways to well-being.

five-ways-to-wellbeing-at-work-toolkit. For more general information on the five ways to well-being, 'Health in Mind' in Scotland has a video explaining each of the five ways https://www.health-in-mind.org.uk/resources/5_ways_to_wellbeing/d140/ and Northern Health in Australia has a short video showing a clear example of all five https://www.5waystowellbeing.org.au/.

Practitioner skills activity 4j: Five ways to well-being.

Look at the resources on the five ways to well-being in the section above and Figure 4.9. How could you promote the five ways to well-being for employees in your place of work or in a place you frequently see people working such as in a supermarket? Think of a different idea for each of the five ways.

ALTERNATIVE SETTINGS FOR HEALTH

There are a variety of alternative settings used to promote health that may not traditionally come to mind when you think of health promotion. Parks, cinemas, nightclubs, pharmacies, laundromats, beauty salons, barbers, cafes, sports centres and convenience stores have all been used as places for health promotion. Below are two examples chosen to illustrate alternative settings. Nightclubs, bars and pubs and barbershops. These spaces represent the community settings of the future as we seek new ways to promote health in those who are excluded from traditional health education approaches.

HEALTHY NIGHTCLUBS, BARS AND PUBS

Nightclubs, bars and pubs have been used for campaigns aimed at being safe. These include 'Designated Driver' (DES) campaigns like https://www.think.gov.uk/campaign/designated-driver/ to reduce drink-driving, 'Ask for Angela', to support women who are on a date that doesn't feel right https://www.lincolnshire.gov.uk/crime-prevention/sexual-violence-abuse/2 and 'The Good Night Out' campaign https://www.goodnightoutcampaign.org/ to prevent sexual harassment and assault. The Good Night Out also encourages venues to change their environments to be more inclusive for example through the provision of gender-neutral toilets https://www.goodnightoutcampaign.org/wp-content/uploads/2021/03/toilets.pdf. At a broader policy level 'Pub watch' is a voluntary scheme to promote safer drinking environments in the UK. Their website has different examples of keeping people safe from across the UK https://www.nationalpubwatch.org.uk/.

HEALTHY BARBERSHOPS

A setting outside the UK is 'barbershops' which have been used in the USA to reach ethnic minority males. Linnan (2019) highlights how barbershops are safe spaces where men gather to talk, play games or watch sports with trusted male role models thus providing a safe environment for health discussions. An example is the 'American Black Barbershop Health Outreach' programme which started in 2006, where barbers screen, educate and refer their customers for specific health conditions like high blood pressure. You can read more about this programme at https://www.blackbarbershop.org/. This model has been expanded on in other areas, for example, HIV risk reduction sessions in barbershops (Wilson et al., 2019).

DEMENTIA-FRIENDLY COMMUNITIES

There are around 55 million people in the world living with dementia (Alzheimers Disease International, 2022) and in the UK, over one-third of people with dementia say they felt lonely recently, and more than one-quarter of carers felt cut off from society (Alzheimer's Society, 2022). Community action can help people live well with dementia and make it easier to navigate community spaces. Alzheimer's Disease International has many resources around dementia and examples of dementia-friendly initiatives from all regions of the world https://www.alzint.org/reports-resources/. Chapter 1 'The field of health promotion' has links to becoming a 'Dementia friend'.

A dementia-friendly community has the potential to improve the quality of life of people affected by dementia (Buckner et al., 2019). Communities work to increase awareness of dementia and modify social and physical environments to increase social connections and reduce stigma. An example is a 'memory café' which provides a café style environment for people living with dementia and their carers and families. They are designed to reduce social isolation, build friendships and give carers and relatives a space to relax. Age UK has a guide to starting a dementia café at https://www.ageuk.org.uk/bp-assets/globalassets/norfolk/age-uk-norfolk-dementia-cafe-toolkit.pdf.

Health promotion in practice example: Environments for people living with dementia.

Sturge et al. (2021) explored how people with dementia see and interact with features of their social and built environments. They found that features of the built environment like shops, clear signage and traffic control measures can support independence and provide social interaction. However, using technology in public spaces such as in a bank, and changes in familiar landscapes such as roadworks, were potentially challenging.

SUPPORTIVE FOOD ENVIRONMENTS

Global challenges affect food at the local level. The Russia–Ukraine conflict as highlighted in Chapter 1 'The field of health promotion', has resulted in disruptions to global food and fuel prices. Globally, as both Russia and Ukraine are major agricultural powers, this also creates challenges for other countries relying on food imports from these countries (Ben Hassen & El Bilali, 2022). Covid-19 supply chain disruptions have also complicated the situation with food prices already increasing before the conflict. This example shows us that food security is a major challenge for everyone and that there are vulnerabilities and challenges in global food systems that need sustainable solutions. The 'rising cost of living' is discussed in more detail in Chapter 1 'The field of health promotion'.

Food environments are the places, spaces and contexts that shape the food we buy, prepare and eat. We engage with different food systems in different contexts to make decisions about our food and drinks. What we decide to eat depends on factors like food access, food availability, income, cooking equipment, cooking skills, time, family and cultural values. Supportive food environments require action across different types of policies. The European Public Health Alliance (2019) gives suggestions for different policy levels that encourage supportive food environments, as well as examples of promising best practices such as the sugar levy (sugar tax) at https://epha.org/living-environments-mapping-food-environments/. See the health promotion in practice example about food policy below.

Health promotion in practice example: Supportive food policy.

Two examples of food policies to promote sustainable food environments are 'food composition' and 'food labelling'. 'Food composition' is about what is in food. This includes banning substances known to be harmful to health such as industrially produced trans-fats which can increase the risk of coronary heart disease (CHD). The campaign 'Replace Trans Fats' aims to eliminate industrially-produced trans-fats from the global food supply. Read more at https://www.who.int/teams/nutrition-and-food-safety/replace-trans-fat. *Mandatory food labelling is when manufacturers put information on food packets giving nutritional content about the product. The UK uses a traffic light labelling system which you can watch a video about on the Food Standards Agency (Food Standards Agency, 2023) website* https://www.food.gov.uk/safety-hygiene/check-the-label.

FOOD INSECURITY

SDG 2 aims to 'end hunger, food insecurity and all forms of malnutrition'. A report by the Food and Agriculture Organisation of the UN (2022) shows that food insecurity is getting worse, meaning more hunger and malnutrition. A report from the World Food Summit in 1996 outlined four dimensions (or pillars) of food security; food availability, food access, food utilisation, and food stability (Food and Agriculture Organisation of the UN, 2008).

- Food availability is having sufficient quantities of regularly available food.
- Food access is the physical and economic resources to get food.
- Food utilisation is the way the body uses food, as well as food hygiene, feeding practice, household distribution of food and food preparation.
- Food stability is all three described dimensions over time, for example, conflict or rising food prices can disrupt the dimensions.

A fifth part has recently been suggested; that of sustainability. Some authors like Guiné et al. (2021) argue that sustainability is an important addition to the four dimensions and should be much more explicit, especially given the focus on sustainability in food systems in SDG 2.

In the UK food security is not spread evenly across the country, and some populations are at higher risk of food insecurity than others. People living on a low income are particularly vulnerable. 'Healthy Start' in England, Wales and Northern Ireland, and 'Best Start' in Scotland provide vouchers (or in Scotland a pre-paid card) to support those on a low income with access to healthy food for young children such as fruit and vegetables and prenatal vitamins. Children living in low-income households are also entitled to free school meals across the UK. For more on Healthy Start and Best Start see https://www.healthystart.nhs.uk/.

Health promotion in practice example: #EndChildFoodPoverty (UK).

The coalition #EndChildFoodPoverty is a coalition to improve low-income children's access to food. In 2020 footballer Marcus Rashford was part of a campaign to provide holiday food vouchers to children receiving free school meals. This extends the provision of free school meals to include the school holidays. The coalition includes different third-sector organisations and businesses campaigning to end child food poverty. You can read more about the campaign here https:// foodfoundation.org.uk/initiatives/endchildfoodpoverty-campaign.

ONLINE FOOD ENVIRONMENTS

Covid-19 has changed the way people in the UK buy food. Nesta (2022) highlights the importance of creating healthy online food environments. They report that 20% of households now buy groceries online and show how fast-food restaurants have now expanded into home delivery markets. They suggest online food environments have the potential to provide opportunities to improve the nation's health. Ideas include:

- Doing more to promote healthy food choices such as allowing people to filter searches by 'low fat' or 'low salt'.
- Giving people suggestions for healthy alternative foods when they shop, such as lower-fat options.
- Make online food shopping more convenient and accessible for everyone, such as making supermarket sites easier to navigate.

Practitioner skills activity 4k: Exploring online food environments.

Have a look at a popular online grocery store or a take-out provider in your country. What sort of things do you think they do to encourage unhealthy food choices? How easy is the site to navigate? Could they do things to encourage healthy choices?

THE CHALLENGES OF HEALTHY SETTINGS

One major challenge is the importance large organisations or governments attach to health. An employer might prioritise productivity or profit over the health and well-being of their workforce. Governments might decide to invest in areas that are health-damaging like fossil fuels. Even when organisations or governments do prioritise health there may be financial or infrastructure challenges. For example in 'healthy schools' programmes research suggests barriers like funding reductions, timetable restrictions or lack of education policies to support schools such as sustainable diets (McHugh et al., 2022).

Access to settings is also unequal. For example, workplace programmes can only improve health in those who are employed, and this may increase health inequalities between those who are employed and those who are not. Some populations are unable to work, for example, those who are long-term sick or those living with a physical or learning disability. These groups might also it difficult to access an alternative setting that could support their health.

Settings are not 'neutral' spaces, and there is an imbalance in status or power. In a workplace, for example, managers might have a reputation for not caring about their workers. They might dictate job roles, pay or conditions and workers may feel have little power to change things. Finding evidence for using settings is also quite hard, especially for non-traditional settings. Collecting and disseminating the work that is already being done will help to develop the healthy settings approach.

SUMMARY

This chapter has explored 'creating supportive environments' using a broad definition that includes the natural and built, social-cultural and political environments. Working in this area should complement strategies to 'developing personal skills', through 'strengthening community action'. This will help us to create supportive, inclusive, and accessible environments that promote health and well-being for all. The chapters so far have focussed on people, communities and places. In the next chapter, we are moving to healthcare, and how healthcare can be reorientated to support everyone.

WIDER READING

ONLINE

The resource 'All Our Health' discussed in 'Chapter 5 Reorientating healthcare services', also includes a free e-learning module on workplace health, https://www.e-lfh.org.uk/programmes/all-our-health/.

The *British Medical Journal* (BMJ) has a series of online articles about 'building healthy communities', https://www.bmj.com/building-healthy-communities.

Public Health England (2019). Health matters: Health and work at https://www.gov.uk/government/publications/health-matters-health-and-work/health-matters-health-and-work.

UK Universities Network Toolkit at https://healthyuniversities.ac.uk/toolkit-and-resources/.

WHO (2018). Healthy islands: Best practices in health promotion in the Pacific, https://www.who.int/publications/i/item/9789290618270.

TEXTBOOKS

Woodhall, J., & Cross, R. (2022). *Essentials of health promotion*. Sage, London. Chapters on Healthy Settings.

LISTENING AND WATCHING

TedX has some talks around healthy cities such as 'Growing Healthy Cities'. Glenn Howells. TEDxBrum at https://www.youtube.com/watch?v=GSxd_qKR38E. 'Let's design healthy cities'. Eric Frijters. TEDxAUCollege at https://www.youtube.com/watch?v=eYBy2O3YI2k.

Dalla Lana School of Public Health (Toronto, Canada) Healthy Cities in the SDG era. Series of lectures focussed on SDGS and Healthy cities. Episode 1 can be found here https://www.youtube.com/watch?v=JiL78QU9zHo.

ADDITIONAL REFERENCES

These are the additional references this chapter has used where electronic links have not been provided in the chapter.

Aked, J., Marks, N., Cordon, C., & Thompson, S. (2008). 5 ways to wellbeing. New Economics Foundation. Available at https://neweconomics.org/2008/10/five-ways-to-wellbeing.

Alzheimer's Society. (2022). Making your community more dementia friendly. Available at https://www.alzheimers.org.uk/get-involved/dementia-friendly-communities.

Alzheimers Disease International. (2022). World Alzheimer Report 2022. Life after diagnosis: Navigating treatment, care and support. Available at https://www.alzint.org/u/World-Alzheimer-Report-2022.pdf.

Ben Hassen, T., & El Bilali, H. (2022). Impacts of the Russia-Ukraine war on global food security: Towards more sustainable and resilient food systems? *Foods*, *11*(15). 10.3390/foods11152301.

Bormet, M., Kishoyian, J., Siame, Y., Ngalande, N., Jr., Erb, K., Parker, K., Huber, D., & Hardee, K. (2021). Faith-based advocacy for family planning works: Evidence from Kenya and Zambia. *Global Health Science and Practice*, *9*(2), 254–263. 10.9745/ghsp-d-20-00641.

Brutus, L., Mackie, P., Millard, A., Fraser, A., Conacher, A., Hardie, S., McDowall, L., & Meechan, H. (2012). *Better health, better lives for prisoners: A framework for improving the health of Scotland's prisoners*. ScotPHN, SHPMG, Scottish Prison Service, Glasgow. Available at https://www.scotphn.net/

wp-content/uploads/2015/10/A-framework-for-improving-the-health-of-Scotlands-prisoners-Volume-1.pdf.

Buckner, S., Darlington, N., Woodward, M., Buswell, M., Mathie, E., Arthur, A., Lafortune, L., Killett, A., Mayrhofer, A., Thurman, J., & Goodman, C. (2019). Dementia friendly communities in England: A scoping study. *International Journal of Geriatric Psychiatry*, *34*(8), 1235–1243. 10.1002/gps.5123.

Criminal Justice Joint Inspection. (2021). A joint thematic inspection of the criminal justice journey for individuals with mental health needs and disorders. Available at https://www.justiceinspectorates.gov.uk/cjji/inspections/mentalhealth2021/.

Department for Education. (2022). Period product scheme for schools and colleges in England. Available at https://www.gov.uk/government/publications/period-products-in-schools-and-colleges/period-product-scheme-for-schools-and-colleges-in-england.

Diendéré, E. A., Traoré, K., Bernatas, J. J., Idogo, O., Dao, A. K., Traoré, G. K., Napon/Zongo, P. D., Ouédraogo/Dioma, S., Bognounou, R., Diallo, I., Ouédraogo/Sondo, A. K., & Niamba, P. A. (2021). Prison health priorities in Burkina Faso: a cross-sectional study in the two largest detention environments in Burkina Faso. *International Journal of Prison Health*. 10.1108/ijph-04-2021-0036.

Dunn, C. G., Wilcox, S., Saunders, R. P., Kaczynski, A. T., Blake, C. E., & Turner-McGrievy, G. M. (2021). Healthy eating and physical activity interventions in faith-based settings: A systematic review using the reach, effectiveness/efficacy, adoption, implementation, maintenance framework. *American Journal of Preventive Medicine*, *60*(1), 127–135. 10.1016/j.amepre.2020.05.014.

European Public Health Alliance. (2019). What are food environments? Available at https://epha.org/what-are-food-environments/.

Faith Action. (2023). Faith action resources. Available at https://www.faithaction.net/our-resources/.

Food and Agriculture Organisation of the UN. (2008). An introduction to the basic concepts of food security. Available at https://www.fao.org/3/al936e/al936e00.pdf.

Food and Agriculture Organization of the United Nations. (2022). The state of food security and nutrition in the world 2022. Available at https://www.fao.org/documents/card/en/c/cc0639en.

Food Standards Agency. (2023). Check the label. Available at https://www.food.gov.uk/safety-hygiene/check-the-label.

Guiné, R. P. F., Pato, M. L. J., Costa, C. A. D., Costa, D., Silva, P., & Martinho, V. (2021). Food security and sustainability: Discussing the four pillars to encompass other dimensions. *Foods*, *10*(11). 10.3390/foods10112732.

International Conference on Health Promoting Universities and Colleges. (2015). Okanagan Charter: An international charter for health promoting universities & colleges. Available at https://open.library.ubc.ca/collections/53926/items/1.0132754.

Langford, R., Bonell, C., Jones, H., Pouliou, T., Murphy, S., Waters, E., Komro, K., Gibbs, L., Magnus, D., & Campbell, R. (2015). The World Health Organization's Health Promoting Schools framework: A Cochrane systematic review and meta-analysis. *BMC Public Health*, *15*, 130. 10.1186/s12889-015-1360-y.

Lewis, J. (2022). Research briefing: Sexual harassment and violence in further and higher education. Available at https://commonslibrary.parliament.uk/research-briefings/cbp-9438/.

Linnan, L. A. (2019). Growing evidence for barbershop-based interventions to promote health and address chronic diseases. *American Journal of Public Health*, *109*(8), 1073–1074. 10.2105/ajph.2019.305182.

McHugh, C., Lloyd, J., Logan, S., & Wyatt, K. (2022). Enablers and barriers English secondary schools face in promoting healthy diet and physical activity behaviours. *Health Promot Int*, *37*(2). 10.1093/heapro/daab148.

Mind. (2023). Mentally healthy universities programme. Available at https://www.mind.org.uk/workplace/mentally-healthy-universities-programme/.

National Institute for Clinical Excellence. (2022a). Mental well-being at work NICE guideline [NG212]. Available at https://www.nice.org.uk/guidance/ng212.

National Institute for Clinical Excellence. (2022b). Reducing sexually transmitted infections. NICE guideline [NG221]. Available at https://www.nice.org.uk/guidance/ng221.

Nesta. (2022). How improving online food environments can support our health. Available at https://www.nesta.org.uk/blog/how-improving-online-food-environments-can-support-our-health/.

Office for Students. (2023). Resources for student safety and wellbeing. Available at https://www.officeforstudents.org.uk/advice-and-guidance/student-wellbeing-and-protection/resources-for-student-safety-and-wellbeing/.

Peterson, J., Atwood, J. R., & Yates, B. (2002). Key elements for church-based health promotion programs: Outcome-based literature review. *Public Health Nursing*, *19*(6), 401–411. 10.1046/j.1525-1446.2002.19602.x.

Public Health England. (2017). Guide to healthy living: Mosques. Available at https://assets.publishing.service.gov.uk/government/uploads/system/uploads/attachment_data/file/619891/Guide_to_Healthy_Living_Mosques.PDF.

Scottish Government. (2019). The National Plan for Scotland's Islands. Available at https://www.gov.scot/publications/national-plan-scotlands-islands/pages/10/.

Sidossis, A., Gaviola, G. C., Sotos-Prieto, M., & Kales, S. (2021). Healthy lifestyle interventions across diverse workplaces: A summary of the current evidence. *Curr Opin Clin Nutr Metab Care*, *24*(6), 490–503. 10.1097/mco.0000000000000794.

Sturge, J., Nordin, S., Sussana Patil, D., Jones, A., Légaré, F., Elf, M., & Meijering, L. (2021). Features of the social and built environment that contribute to the well-being of people with dementia who live at home: A scoping review. *Health & Place*, *67*, 102483. 10.1016/j.healthplace.2020. 102483.

The Health Foundation. (2022). Evidence hub. Available at https://www. health.org.uk/evidence-hub.

Tomalin, E., Sadgrove, J., & Summers, R. (2019). Health, faith and therapeutic landscapes: Places of worship as Black, Asian and Minority Ethnic (BAME) public health settings in the United Kingdom. *Social Science & Medicine*, *230*, 57–65. 10.1016/j.socscimed.2019.03.006.

UK Government. (2023). Prisons and probation. Available at https://www. gov.uk/browse/justice/prisons-probation.

United Nations. (2015). Sustainable development goals. Available at https:// sdgs.un.org/goals.

United Nations. (2023). Nelson Mandela rules. Available at https://www.un. org/en/events/mandeladay/mandela_rules.shtml.

United Nations Office on Drugs and Crime. (2015). The United Nations standard minimum rules for the treatment of prisoners (the Nelson Mandela Rules). Available at https://www.unodc.org/documents/justice-and-prison-reform/Nelson_Mandela_Rules-E-ebook.pdf.

Universities UK. (2023). Publications. Available at https://www.universitiesuk. ac.uk/what-we-do/policy-and-research/publications?topic=42.

Van Hout, M. C., & Mhlanga-Gunda, R. (2019). Prison health situation and health rights of young people incarcerated in sub-Saharan African prisons and detention centres: A scoping review of extant literature. *BMC International Health and Human Rights*, *19*(1), 17. 10.1186/s12914-019-0200-z.

Waterworth, C., & Thorpe, A. (2017). Applying the Okanagan Charter in Aotearoa New Zealand. *JANZSSA - Journal of the Australian and New Zealand Student Services Association*, *25*(1). Available at https://janzssa.scholasticahq. com/article/1338-applying-the-okanagan-charter-in-aotearoa-new-zealand.

Wilson, T. E., Gousse, Y., Joseph, M. A., Browne, R. C., Camilien, B., McFarlane, D., Mitchell, S., Brown, H., Urraca, N., Romeo, D., Johnson, S., Salifu, M., Stewart, M., Vavagiakis, P., & Fraser, M. (2019). HIV prevention for Black heterosexual men: The barbershop talk with brothers cluster randomized trial. *American Journal of Public Health*, *109*(8), 1131–1137. 10.2105/ajph.2019.305121.

Wirth, T., Peters, C., Nienhaus, A., & Schablon, A. (2021). Interventions for workplace violence prevention in emergency departments: A systematic review. *International Journal of Environmental Research and Public Health*, *18*(16). 10.3390/ijerph18168459.

Woodall, J., & Freeman, C. (2021). Developing health and wellbeing in prisons: An analysis of prison inspection reports in Scotland. *BMC Health Services Research*, *21*(1), 314. 10.1186/s12913-021-06337-z.

World Economic Forum. (2021). Healthy cities and communities playbook. A white paper by the World Economic Forum's Platform for Shaping the Future of Consumption. Available at https://www3.weforum.org/docs/WEE_Healthy_Cities_Communities_Playbook_2021.pdf.

World Health Organization. (1986). The Ottawa charter for health promotion: First international conference on health promotion, Ottawa, 21 November 1986. Available at https://www.who.int/teams/health-promotion/enhanced-wellbeing/first-global-conference.

World Health Organization. (2015). 2015 Yanuca Island Declaration on health in Pacific island countries and territories: Eleventh Pacific Health Ministers Meeting, 15–17 April 2015. Available at https://www.who.int/publications/i/item/PHMM_declaration_2015.

World Health Organization. (2021). Making every school a health-promoting school – Implementation Guidance. Available at https://www.who.int/publications/i/item/9789240025073.

World Health Organization. (2022). Drinking water. Available at https://www.who.int/news-room/fact-sheets/detail/drinking-water.

World Health Organization. (2023). Status report on prison health in the WHO European Region 2022. Available at https://www.who.int/europe/publications/i/item/9789289058674.

World Prison Brief. (2023). Ten country prisons project. Available at https://www.prisonstudies.org/ten-country-prisons-project.

5

REORIENTATING HEALTH SERVICES

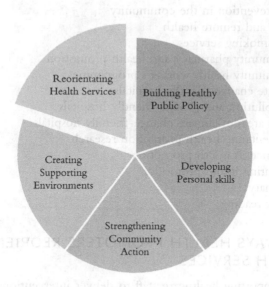

Figure 5.1 Reorientating health services.

DOI: 10.4324/9781003462323-6

- Five ways health promoters reorientate health services
- Overview
- Health professions and health promotion
- All our health
- Making every contact count (MECC)
- Social prescribing
- Examples of social prescribing in England, Northern Ireland, Scotland and Wales.
- Inclusion healthcare
- Homelessness and healthcare
- Inclusive healthcare spaces
- Cultural safety
- Reducing harm from healthcare
- Antimicrobial stewardship
- Medication management and deprescribing
- Anchor institutions
- Fall prevention in the community
- Rural and remote health
- Stop smoking services
- Community pharmacy and health promotion
- Community health worker's programmes
- Climate change-friendly hospitals
- Air pollution and climate-friendly hospitals
- Seven areas of climate change-friendly hospitals
- Reorientating health promotion research
- Evidence in health promotion
- Evaluating health promotion
- Summary
- Wider reading

FIVE WAYS HEALTH PROMOTERS REORIENTATE HEALTH SERVICES

(1) Supporting healthcare staff to deliver interventions for behaviour change in areas like alcohol or physical activity.

(2) Training a wide variety of healthcare workers such as pharmacists or dentists to provide services such as smoking cessation.

(3) Advocating for stewardship of resources such as antimicrobials.
(4) Finding ways to change healthcare or challenge healthcare practices to ensure they are inclusive to those who need care the most.
(5) Promoting or delivering 'social prescribing' in community settings (Figure 5.1).

OVERVIEW

The health sector in the UK is slowly evolving from a treatment and curative service to a service that focusses on prevention. There are two types of prevention:

- **Primary prevention:** This type of prevention is to stop people from getting sick in the first place by reducing risks. Sun safety campaigns try to do this as they try to prevent sunburn and the risk of skin cancer.
- **Secondary prevention:** With this type of prevention someone already has a health problem. The idea is to stop something from getting worse or support people to get better. An example is supporting people living with diabetes with lifestyle modifications to prevent further health complications.

The NHS long-term plan (NHS, 2019) has a strong focus on both types of prevention. For example, it says that every person who is admitted to a hospital that smokes will be offered NHS-funded stop-smoking support (secondary prevention). It also says it will continue to try and reduce obesity by providing healthy foods for all staff, patients and the public (primary prevention).

A move to prevention challenges the way many people think about healthcare. We have to think about health from the perspective of the whole person and their social, physical and mental health needs. It requires recognition that health is socially determined and that if we only focus on the presenting medical condition, we are ignoring the daily circumstances in which people live their lives. To do this we need changes across the whole of the health sector. We need to improve how we interact and engage with people and communities to support their health. We also need to make sure those who need healthcare are getting good quality care, and that no one gets left out.

See the example below that shows the different ways we can reorientate healthcare.

Health promotion in practice example: Ethnicity and mental health project (England)

The ethnicity and mental health improvement project (EMHIP) in Wandsworth (London, UK) is designed to reduce ethnic inequalities in access, experience and outcome of mental health care. Their project works in five ways. This includes creating mental health and well-being hubs in the community, for example with places of worship. They also aim to increase their mental health service options, reduce restrictive and coercive practices, and ensure a culturally capable workforce. For more information, including an example of a well-being hub in a place of worship see https://emhip.co.uk/.

HEALTH PROFESSIONS AND HEALTH PROMOTION

Some health professions have an explicit health promotion and public health remit. For example, in the UK many School Nurses and Health Visitors complete a 'specialist community public health nursing' course. School nurses deliver services for children and young people in education settings. You can read more about school nursing practice in a toolkit at https://www.rcn.org.uk/professional-development/publications/pub-007320. A health visitor works with young children and their families in the community. See more at https://ihv.org.uk/families/what-is-a-hv/. To read more on health services that support children and young people including midwifery and health visiting see https://www.gov.uk/government/publications/commissioning-of-public-health-services-for-children. Chapter 3 'Strengthening community action' also has more on community health workers in low-income countries who also have a preventive health role.

Other health professions have much potential to offer health promotion in their daily work. These include physiotherapists, occupational therapists, opticians, audiologists, dentists, pharmacists, doctors, nurses and midwives. It is not just health professionals that can offer health promotion advice, guidance or deliver programmes.

Many other types of workers can also deliver health promotion or health education from teachers and social workers to sport and leisure staff and housing officers. 'All Our Health' (Public Health England, 2019a) is a resource to encourage different health professionals to engage in health promotion and health education in their daily work. This is discussed below.

'ALL OUR HEALTH'

The Office for Health Improvement and Disparities 'All Our Health' policy (Public Health England, 2019a) is a health promotion and illness prevention framework with resources for healthcare practitioners. NHS Health Education for England and eLearning for Healthcare (Elfh) have developed a wide range of virtual resources and as I write (in 2023) there are 33 e-learning sessions from air pollution and alcohol to healthy ageing and healthy workplaces. There are also sections around health inequalities and inclusion in healthcare. Most e-learning modules contain videos or animations, and four sections: Why does it matter? What can I do to help? Where can I find information? And a knowledge check. See more at https://www.e-lfh.org.uk/programmes/all-our-health/.

MAKING EVERY CONTACT COUNT (MECC)

Making every contact count (MECC) is an opportunistic way to promote healthy lifestyles between patients and healthcare practitioners on a day-to-day basis. It suggests that people working in different sectors such as healthcare, voluntary organisations or local authorities should offer healthy lifestyle information to everyone and 'start conversations' about health. Training is available to anyone without registration and includes how to have a conversation with others, and signposting to services. You can read more or do the training for free at https://www.e-lfh.org.uk/programmes/making-every-contact-count/. Anyone can be involved with MECC, but healthcare practitioners are ideally placed to support people. For example, dentists could deliver advice on oral cancer, oral hygiene, tobacco or alcohol. See an example of a prevention toolkit for dental teams at https://www.gov.uk/government/publications/delivering-better-oral-health-an-evidence-based-toolkit-for-prevention.

SOCIAL PRESCRIBING

Social prescribing uses a non-medical (meaning no drugs or medicine) option to improve health. Social prescribing is a type of community referral where a practitioner, typically a healthcare professional refers a person to a 'link worker'. The link worker then explores the issues that the person is facing and finds the right services to support them. A medical consultation with a GP (General Practitioner) cannot always address the factors that contribute to poor health outcomes such as financial problems, social isolation difficulties or living with a health problem over a long period. Torjesen (2016) cites evidence that around 20% of GP consultations are for a problem that is primarily a social problem, rather than a medical problem. For example, living in damp housing is linked to increased respiratory problems. A person may present with a respiratory problem to a health professional, but the primary cause of the problem is poor housing. The National Academy for Social Prescribing has created two short videos that give a clear overview of social prescribing on its website https://socialprescribingacademy.org.uk/about-us/what-is-social-prescribing/.

Practitioner skills activity 5a: What would you socially prescribe?

Imagine that you are working as a social prescriber. Jessy comes to see you. She is 22 years old and has depression and anxiety. She has been unemployed for three years after the factory she was working in closed. She left school at 16 with few qualifications. She lives with her mum in a small flat in a town. She is a carer for her mum who had a stroke three years ago. She does not go out much as she doesn't like leaving her mum alone at home. What type of services or support could you socially prescribe for Jessy?

Most social prescribing schemes involve a range of activities that are provided by different voluntary or community organisations. They include activities such as art and craft, gardening, physical activity or peer support schemes. A more detailed overview of social prescribing with examples is available from the King's Fund website https://www.kingsfund.org.uk/publications/social-prescribing.

EXAMPLES OF SOCIAL PRESCRIBING IN ENGLAND, NORTHERN IRELAND, SCOTLAND AND WALES

- The Bromley-by-Bow centre in England is one of the first places to use a social prescribing approach. The centre was first a 'Healthy Living Centre' in 1997 and has continued to offer a range of services linked to health, employment, education and other areas that centre on a holistic view of health and well-being. A BBC film has been made about the centre which you can watch at https://www.bbbc.org.uk/social-prescribing/.
- The IMPACTAgewell® programme in Mid and East Antrim (Northern Ireland) is for those over 60 living and is linked with GP practices in the area. Types of support include befriending, energy efficiency checks, benefits advice, lunch clubs and art/history clubs. https://www.meaap.co.uk/impactagewell/.
- A charity working with people who have, or are at risk of having, lifelong health conditions in Lorn and Oban (Scotland). They work to support people to learn the skills and tools to self-manage their health through two programmes; ADAPT for people who require specialist support or who are newly diagnosed and THRIVE, for support with self-management and adaptation of healthy behaviours. https://www.lornhealthyoptions.co.uk/.
- To reduce isolation and loneliness in the Aneurin Bevan Health Board (Wales) the scheme 'Ffrind I Mi/Friend of Mine' has been designed to connect people across Wales. You can read more here https://www.ffrindimi.co.uk/.

Social prescribing originated in the UK, but more recently other countries have created national hubs or are discussing the merits of this approach. One example is in Canada where a hub has been created to share good practices and connect people to community support by the Canadian Institute for Social Prescribing (CISP), https://www.socialprescribing.ca/.

INCLUSION HEALTHCARE

Inclusion healthcare is a term used to describe the process of making sure those who are socially excluded can access and get the services

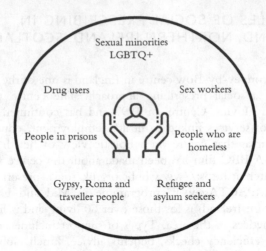

Figure 5.2 Inclusion health care.

they need. Someone who is socially excluded can experience poorer health both through barriers to healthcare and through multiple risk factors for poor health. Figure 5.2 shows the population groups most likely to be excluded from healthcare services.

Figure 5.2 shows those most likely to be excluded include those who are homeless, drug users, those in prisons, sex workers, refugees and asylum seekers, migrants, Gypsy, Roma and traveller populations or sexual minorities (LGBTQ+). See Chapter 3 'Strengthening community action' for more on including everyone in community work. Making healthcare available to everyone means we need to:

• Understand how social exclusion influences healthcare access and use,
• Develop skills and services that can support people's health and well-being better

Practitioner skills activity 5b: Outreach health promotion.
Look at Figure 5.2. Which socially excluded groups might benefit from one or more of these interventions?

- *Vaccine delivery in community centres or libraries.*
- *Non-judgemental sexual health services located in large shopping centres.*
- *Community education initiatives that tell people about their healthcare entitlements.*
- *Needle exchange programmes for substance misuse in town centres.*
- *Blood pressure monitoring checks in temporary accommodation settings.*

Many healthcare interventions offer big benefits to those who experience challenges accessing healthcare. For example, offering methadone for treating opioid dependency such as heroin addiction, providing direct observational therapy (DOTs) for those living with HIV or tuberculosis (TB), or providing safe injecting sites to reduce high-risk needle sharing in drug users (Luchenski et al., 2018). If people cannot access or use these healthcare services this puts these populations at risk of preventable death or harm.

The resource 'All Our Health' mentioned earlier in this chapter suggests ways practitioners can work so that everyone can access the services they need. These include being familiar with what people are entitled to, finding ways to help people attend appointments, and finding out about what support services can help the people. See the example below on supporting those with a learning disability.

Health promotion in practice example: Mencap 'Treat me well' and 'Hospital passports' (UK).

The Mencap 'Treat me well' campaign is a campaign to try and change how the NHS treats people with a learning disability in hospital. The campaign calls on NHS staff to make reasonable adjustments for people with a learning disability including better communication, more time and more information. The website also provides a 'Hospital passport' resource These passports tell the hospital about the person living with a learning disability, their healthcare, their learning disability, how they like to communicate and how to make things easier for them. You can read more at https://www.mencap.org.uk/get-involved/campaign-mencap/treat-me-well.

HOMELESSNESS AND HEALTHCARE

Those who are homeless experience some of the worst health outcomes in the UK. The term 'Homeless' includes those people

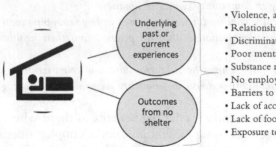

Figure 5.3 Homelessness and health.

sleeping rough, using emergency or temporary accommodation as well as short-term stays with friends or family, known as 'sofa surfing'. The average age of death of someone homeless in 2020 was 45.9 for men and 41.6 for women (Office of National Statistics, 2021a). For comparison, the average life expectancy in the UK is over 30 years more at 79.0 years for men and 82.9 for women (Office of National Statistics, 2021b). Being homeless means much more than simply not having a house. Figure 5.3 highlights some of the risks of homelessness on health.

Figure 5.3 shows that those who are homeless are more likely to have poorer physical and mental health, which can lead to multiple morbidities and a higher risk of premature death. Health can be a cause and a consequence of homelessness. For example, an inability to work due to poor mental or physical health means no money to pay for accommodation (a cause), but both mental and physical health can be worsened through homelessness (a consequence). Being homeless also increases the risk of exposure to risk factors for illness. For example, the risk of infectious disease is increased through sharing facilities like bedrooms in temporary accommodation, the lack of publicly available washrooms and underlying medical conditions or substance use disorders which may encourage disease transmission, for example, needle sharing (Mosites et al., 2022).

Health promotion in practice example: Experiences of people who are homeless.
A peer research project in Birmingham identified significant barriers to accessing healthcare services including travel costs, cost of mobile phone credit,

inflexible appointment systems or long waiting times. Read more at #healthnow (Groundswell & Crisis, 2021). Groundswell UK also have the 'listen up!' hub that collects homeless experiences from trained community reporters using mobile phones to document stories. Read more at https://groundswell-listenup-hub.org/.

Many health and care services fail to meet the needs of people sleeping rough as they are not set up to meet the complex needs of homeless people (Crisis UK, 2022). Cream (2020) suggests that services are often set up in the way that they are because many of us have never experienced homelessness and the multiple struggles over safety, food, and shelter and the impact of these on our health. They argue that health needs are closely connected to housing needs and solutions do not just rest with healthcare, but with joined-up service working that include local authorities, and voluntary organisations. Currently, healthcare services and housing services are two quite separate services, and a joined-up approach is required to meet the needs of those who are homeless. Read more about delivering healthcare for people who sleep rough at https://www.kingsfund.org.uk/publications/delivering-health-care-people-sleep-rough.

INCLUSIVE HEALTHCARE SPACES

To make spaces more inclusive, we need to reorientate our practitioner skills, modify the settings we deliver care, and change organisational practices so policies support fair care. This three-tiered approach to inclusion healthcare is demonstrated in Figure 5.4.

Figure 5.4 shows the three tiers where health promoters can advocate, enable and mediate change. These are at the individual level, the healthcare settings level (the clinic, health centre or service delivery space), and the healthcare organisation level. These are discussed below.

Training healthcare workers is often recommended to improve knowledge, attitude and self-confidence in addressing the health needs of socially excluded groups. For example, research consistently shows training practitioners using programmes designed to promote LGBTQ+ competency can increase knowledge and

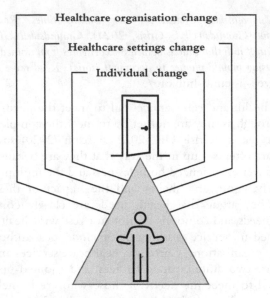

Figure 5.4 Three tiers of inclusion healthcare.

promote more accepting attitudes (Bristol et al., 2018). Everyone who uses healthcare should feel welcome and safe. People may access healthcare in times of stress or anxiety and the waiting room in a clinic or health centre can be a space that people find uncomfortable (Kearns et al., 2020). Settings could have statements of equality telling people everyone is welcome, welcome messages in different languages or posters of what's on locally to support health. Settings should have inclusive facilities like easy disabled access, breastfeeding facilities or gender-neutral bathroom spaces.

Health promotion in practice example: The value of health to those who are homeless.

Research exploring women and homelessness in Sweden found that women highly valued healthcare during times of homelessness (Kneck et al., 2022). Core values included being treated with respect and feeling safe and secure when seeking care. Discussion is framed using a model of 'do something, do more, do better'. Do something includes listening to women, do more includes removing barriers, and do better includes delivering joined-up care across different sectors and services to support women who are homeless.

In the UK, the Equality Act 2010 (Government Equalities Office, 2010) legally means that people with protected characteristics cannot be discriminated against. All healthcare organisations should have clear equality and discrimination policies in place and healthcare practitioners should know what they mean for their practice. Some employers work to get inclusion awards. For example, the Stonewall Health Equality Index (Stonewall UK, 2023) shows employers understand their LGBTQ+ employee experiences and demonstrate a commitment to change. You can read more about this here https://www.stonewall.org.uk/creating-inclusive-workplaces/workplace-equality-indices/uk-workplace-equality-index.

CULTURAL SAFETY

Cultural awareness and cultural safety are not the same things. Cultural awareness is about understanding that there may be cultural differences between people. It is about understanding that different cultural groups may have different illness beliefs and interpretations, different factors that discourage health-seeking behaviours, or different cultural practices that may be commonly used to promote health and prevent sickness. See the migrant women example below.

Health promotion in practice example: Migrant women and maternal health services (EU).

Research on migrant women accessing maternal health services in the EU by (Fair et al., 2020) identified the variety of difficulties women faced accessing care in unfamiliar systems. This includes a lack of knowledge about how the systems work and what they were entitled to, difficulties in accessing care (i.e. registration) and booking or attending appointments (i.e. costs, booking systems). Women also reported needs outside the traditional maternity services remit including difficulties with accommodation, financial struggles and a high burden of loneliness.

'Cultural safety' is a term that is not just about being 'culturally aware' but about also being culturally safe. The concept has come from the colonial context of New Zealand and was introduced to nursing education in the 1990s as a way to try and address power imbalances in healthcare and reduce health inequalities experienced by indigenous peoples (Papps & Ramsden, 1996). It is usually used in the context of ethnic minorities or indigenous population groups.

Healthcare practitioners can make health inequalities worse when they do not recognise the importance of 'power' structures across society and do not think critically about their own dominant culture and cultural systems (Curtis et al., 2019). When we work in health we must reflect on our attitudes and beliefs about others. This includes thinking about the way history, society and politics continue to shape health and healthcare today. This will help us to be more flexible in how we support people who are different to us (Urbanoski et al., 2020). This may be an uncomfortable process, as we have to face up to how we can be judgemental or discriminatory against people who are different. See the practitioner skills activity below.

Practitioner skills activity 5c: Being culturally safe.

Who are the indigenous people or ethnic minority populations in your country or city? What is the impact of historical events like colonialism, segregation or discrimination on their health? Has this meant that their language, history, culture or knowledge is seen as less important? What could this mean for their health today?

A good health promoter is a culturally safe health promoter. Remember that some people are not seeking healthcare or getting what they need as they do not have the 'power' to do so or do not know what they are entitled to have. They may have experienced a history of discrimination, racism, trauma, violence or marginalisation which stops them from feeling safe in a healthcare environment. They may disengage from care that is unfamiliar, not know how to seek the right care or find it difficult to speak about what they need. We need to make safe spaces that are inclusive for all in our health promotion work and find ways to include everyone. See Chapter 3 'Strengthening community action' for more on 'power'.

REDUCING HARM FROM HEALTHCARE

Reorientating healthcare services include reducing harm from healthcare interventions such as treatments or medications. We often assume that a hospital is the best place for someone to be, but some people may become more unwell when they go to the hospital. Preventable death and disability among those who have a hospital stay include healthcare-acquired infections such as methicillin-resistant *Staphylococcus aureus* (MRSA) and *Clostridium difficile* (*C. difficile*). Some people have poorer experiences from being in hospitals. For example, people living with a learning disability can experience distress or anxiety and people who need a hospital stay are also more likely to experience reduced mobility. Older people in particular are at high risk of negative outcomes from reduced mobility, and services exist across the UK to try and keep older people out of hospitals. Examples include home adaption interventions or fall prevention programmes to reduce emergency fall admissions or offering out-of-hours clinical services such as falls and frailty response teams. See also the health promotion in practice example of Welsh Ambulance Service Trust fall response service later in this chapter.

ANTIMICROBIAL STEWARDSHIP

The UK government has a 20-year vision, and a five-year national action plan for how it will tackle Antimicrobial Resistance (AMR) by 2040 (Department of Health and Social Care, 2019). The plan includes reducing drug-resistant infections, reducing the use of antimicrobials, and preventing healthcare-acquired infections. Antimicrobials are needed in healthcare for the prevention of ill-health and curative purposes. Over-use or incorrect use can lead to AMR meaning people are at risk of currently preventable disease.

Practitioner skills activity 5d: Antimicrobial stewardship.

Have you ever been unwell and been given medication to help you get better? Did you follow all the instructions that you were given about when to take the medicine and how much to take? Have you ever taken antibiotics or antimicrobials that were not prescribed by a healthcare practitioner? Do you know where antibiotics are used outside of healthcare?

Antimicrobial stewardship is an approach to preserving the effectiveness of antimicrobials by looking after them. National Institute of Clinical Excellence (2015) guidance suggests a combination of interventions including a political commitment to prioritise AMR, monitoring drug use, changing health prescribing decisions and educating people on the use of antimicrobials. The UK Health Security Agency has a video about antimicrobial resistance: What does it mean, and why does it matter at this link https://www.youtube.com/channel/UCoFX8yfaEwXNEu3HgLdfomQ

Health promotion in practice example: Reducing antimicrobial resistance (AMR) globally

'World antimicrobial awareness week' aims to increase knowledge and best practice of AMR. See more at https://www.who.int/campaigns/world-antimicrobial-awareness-week. There is a wide range of actions that are promoted through this week. This includes pledging to be an 'antibiotic guardian' at https://antibioticguardian.com/. See more resources including how to set up a knowledge cafe at https://www.gov.uk/government/collections/european-antibiotic-awareness-day-resources.

MEDICATION MANAGEMENT AND DEPRESCRIBING

Around 10% of medications are over-prescribed (Department of Health and Social Care, 2021). This means that patients may experience harm through taking medication. There are also extra costs to healthcare if a medicine is given that is not needed. Deprescribing is a way of reviewing, reducing or discontinuing medications that may cause potential harm. It can use technology to review prescriptions and explore alternatives to medicines. Commonly, deprescribing is the process of identifying patients with severe co-morbidities (meaning multiple health problems), significant functional decline or polypharmacy (using multiple drugs at once). Drugs are identified for deprescribing and then reduced or withdrawn over a specific time frame known as a tapering schedule. Toolkits such as the STOPP-Start toolkit is a screening tool that can help identify people who might be appropriate for a medication review and suggests the right treatment(s) (O'Mahony et al., 2015). Alternatives may be considered with individuals to support self-management of conditions. See the case study on living with pain as an example below.

Health promotion in practice example: Living with pain.

People living with pain may take medication for long periods that may no longer continue to offer benefits. Examples of alternative treatment options include self-management programmes or physical activity. NHS Inform (Scotland) (2021) has a self-help guide for people living with mild to moderate mental health issues to help manage chronic pain. This is an interactive, easy-to-follow guide available at https://www.nhsinform.scot/illnesses-and-

conditions/mental-health/mental-health-self-help-guides/chronic-pain-self-help-guide. *The pain toolkit is for people living around the world with persistent pain and the healthcare workers who support them. It offers pain tools to self-manage pain, online workshops and an online café. See more at* https://www.paintoolkit.org/.

ANCHOR INSTITUTIONS

There are a large number of locations that can be utilised for preventive work. Chapter 4 'Creating supportive environments' has discussed many of the settings such as schools and workplaces that offer opportunities to promote health and may reduce the need for healthcare. Other organisations can also be mobilised to be part of prevention work. Some large organisations like universities and manufacturing businesses have significant infrastructures in a local area as well as resources that could support community health. These organisations are sometimes called 'anchor' institutions.

Anchor institutions have a range of assets such as training or employment opportunities, buildings or land. In the UK, the NHS is an 'anchor institution' (The Health Foundation, 2019). The NHS is situated in local communities, and it is the UK's biggest employer. It owns buildings and land, purchases around 27 billion pounds worth of goods and services each year and can promote innovations, for example by showing practical ways to stay well or by role-modelling a climate change-friendly institution.

Practitioner skills activity 5e: Anchor institutions.
Think about where you live, and what organisations or businesses might have resources, space or opportunities to support health promotion in your community?

These could be used to support health from upskilling local communities into employment, to offering community spaces for meetings or events. Local healthcare settings outside of primary care may also provide a role in supporting communities. Below is an example of 'Merseyside life rooms'.

Health promotion in practice example: Merseyside life rooms (UK).
'The life rooms' is a free NHS service providing spaces for people to meet and learn about resources for their health and well-being. It also provides access

to vocational training, short courses and social activities. It serves Liverpool and Sefton (England) and aims to improve mental and physical well-being for anyone living in this area. The website also has podcasts and A-Z of positive mental health. You can see more at https://www.liferooms.org/.

FALL PREVENTION IN THE COMMUNITY

Falls are the second leading cause of death due to unintentional injuries after road injuries (World Health Organization, 2021a). In the UK around one in three adults aged over 65 and over will fall at least once a year (Office for Health Improvement and Disparities, 2022). Falls harm older people as they can cause injury and death. They also impact people's independence and quality of life. For example, some people who fall may worry they will fall again, or an injury may impact someone's day-to-day living. Reducing falls in the community will reduce emergency hospital admissions, reduce fractures from falls and improve healthy life expectancy for those at risk. Most fall prevention interventions for older adults that live in the community show some level of cost-effectiveness with more value for money in those who are older and at the highest risk (Pinheiro et al., 2022).

Preventing falls requires different types of interventions as people who fall have different risk factors and situations. A fall in the home could be prevented through home modifications, regular sight and hearing testing, medication reviews or exercise programmes including strength and balance training. The consequences of falls can be lessened by reducing risks such as osteoporosis through the provision of Vitamin D supplements. These can reduce the risk of fracture by strengthening bones. Finding quicker ways of reaching those who had a fall can also reduce the negative consequences of a long lie on the floor and allow prompt medical treatment if required. The World Health Organization (2021b) resource 'Step Safely' offers evidence-based strategies for fall prevention across the life course at https://www.who.int/publications/i/item/978924002191-4.

Health promotion in practice example: Welsh Ambulance Service Trust falls response service.

Not everyone who has a fall and calls the emergency services is injured or needs to be admitted to the hospital. In 2018 the Welsh Ambulance Service

Trust and the Aneurin Bevan University Health Board implemented a falls response service to prevent the risk of further harm caused by a long period spent on the floor waiting for an ambulance. Fallers may have one of three responses when they call emergency services. For non-injury falls they are supported by a trained falls assistant. For injury falls, they are assessed by a paramedic and a physiotherapist or occupational therapist.⁻ They are either taken to the hospital, or support is given to prevent the need for avoidable hospital admission and to ensure they can safely remain in their home. For more information see https://www.csp.org.uk/innovations/falls-response-service-multidisciplinary-response-999-falls *and* https://www.gov.wales/written-statement-update-welsh-ambulance-services-nhs-trust-wast-falls-assistants-response-pilot.

RURAL AND REMOTE HEALTH

Rural and remote areas generally have poorer healthcare access, and experience shortages of staff and resources more than urban areas. Infrastructures and services such as the provision of telecommunications like the internet may be absent or unreliable. Journey times to healthcare clinics or hospitals may be long and difficult. Remote health centres may not have the specialist care or equipment that is needed to treat illness. This means creative solutions are needed to support those delivering care, and those seeking care. The Rural Health Information Hub has a disease prevention toolkit that discusses the challenges and strengths of rural health as well as guidance on action at https://www.ruralhealthinfo.org/toolkits/health-promotion.

Telehealth and telemedicine are ways to deliver healthcare through technology such as mobile phones. This might be remote monitoring of health for example the NHS England 'Managing heart failure @ home' at https://www.england.nhs.uk/nhs-at-home/managing-heart-failure-at-home/. It can also be consultations, or specialist care delivered through technology remotely. An example of a Telehealth service for Veterans (USA) can be seen here https://www.youtube.com/watch?v=N5oe5pB7V2g&t=65s. Innovations like virtual wards lend themselves to rural health. A virtual ward aims to deliver hospital-level care in the home through technology. This reduces the need to go to a hospital when unwell and allows people to remain in their homes whilst being closely monitored. See more including videos and resources on how they work in the UK at https://www.england.nhs.uk/virtual-wards/.

Health promotion in practice example: 'Seafit' for fisherman (UK).

'Seafit' is a fisherman's health programme that brings health services to the quayside where fishermen work. They offer health screening and health checks, as well as health education, dentistry and physiotherapy in conjunction with local health services. Services also include 'Shout', a mental health text-messaging service. See more at https://seahospital.org.uk/help-for-you/the-seafit-programme/.

Making use of other healthcare services can also support rural communities. For example, in the UK targeted pharmacy care is an intervention that provides monetary support to rural pharmacies, which if they closed, would disadvantage the local population. The NHS community pharmacist consultation service (CPCS) in NHS England allows patients to have a same-day appointment with a pharmacist for a minor illness or urgent supply of regular medication. You can see more about this, including videos and a case study at https://www.england.nhs.uk/primary-care/pharmacy/pharmacy-integration-fund/community-pharmacist-consultation-service/. The section below also talks more about community pharmacy and health promotion.

Health promotion in practice example: 'On Feirm Ground' (Ireland).

'On Feirm Ground' is a men's health programme in Ireland led by the Men's Development Network. It uses farmers' existing networks of agricultural advisers. Advisers work with farmers on issues connected to farming such as managing their business. Since 2021, training has started to give agriculture advisers more skills to talk to farmers about their health and well-being. See more at https://mensnetwork.ie/ofg/.

Given the challenges of rural communities are often shared across countries, there are many global resources that practitioners can use. The Public Health England (2017) resource on 'health and well-being in rural areas' has a wide variety of rural healthcare studies at https://www.local.gov.uk/sites/default/files/documents/1.39_Health%20in%20rural%20areas_WEB.pdf. The organisation 'Practical Action' has global examples of rural health projects in agricultural communities at https://practicalaction.org/our-aims/farming-that-works/ and this video discusses projects to bring healthcare to rural India at 'Bringing High-Tech Healthcare to India's Poor' https://www.youtube.com/watch?v=0_GxWVZB5HU. The Australia-based 'Journal of Rural and Remote Health' is also a key resource for innovations and interventions for rural health across the healthcare field. See more at https://www.rrh.org.au/.

COMMUNITY PHARMACY AND HEALTH PROMOTION

Community pharmacies have a presence in communities across the globe and those working in them have a key role to play in prevention. Pharmacies are usually locally situated and have the potential to deliver a wide range of services around health and well-being. They do not require appointments and are open at times when access to other healthcare services might be closed. Many currently offer support and information for common illnesses such as eye infections and may offer other services such as needle exchange programmes or stop-smoking support.

A review of pharmacy interventions suggests positive outcomes have been reported for a range of interventions such as smoking services, weight management, vaccination delivery and needle exchange programmes (Thomson et al., 2019). There is also potential for more preventive work within pharmacies. For example, routine health education could be delivered to those collecting prescriptions for conditions such as cardiopulmonary disease (COPD) who smoke tobacco.

Work in many countries suggests that community pharmacists have the capacity and ability to deliver health promotion and education in areas like child health in Ethiopia (Ayele et al., 2022) but that they may not be included in health systems in that country, for example in Brazil community pharmacies are often a first point of access for health care, but their Government stated remit is to only dispense medicines and other health products (Melo et al., 2021) representing a missed opportunity for engagement in health promotion.

Practitioner skills activity 5f: What does your pharmacy offer?

Locate one of your local pharmacies and see what health and wellness services they offer. In England, you can try the 'find a pharmacy' NHS resource https://www.nhs.uk/Service-Search/pharmacy/find-a-pharmacy *in Wales 111 at* https://111.wales.nhs.uk/LocalServices/Default.aspx?s=Pharmacy *and in Scotland NHS inform* https://www.nhsinform.scot/scotlands-service-directory/pharmacies/ *and in Northern Ireland* https://hscbusiness.hscni.net/services/2286.htm. *Other countries may offer a similar service, for example, Australia* https://www.findapharmacy.com.au/.

STOP SMOKING SERVICES

Smoking is a leading cause of preventable illness and death globally killing more than 8 million people a year through the direct act of smoking or exposure to second-hand smoke (WHO, 2022). In the UK, data suggests that about half of all lifelong smokers will die prematurely losing on average approximately 10 years of life (Public Health England, 2019b). Stopping smoking can reduce preventable illness and health care use. The relationship between tobacco and health is well known, and some of the impacts of tobacco on health are shown in Figure 5.5.

Figure 5.5. shows that tobacco smoking impacts nearly every part of the body. It causes around seven of every ten lung cancers, as well as cancers in many parts of the body. It damages the heart and

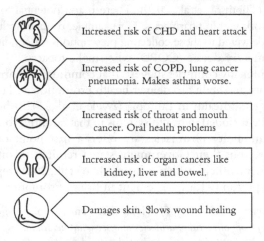

Figure 5.5 Tobacco and how it impacts health.

increases the risk of conditions such as coronary heart disease, stroke, and heart attack. It affects the lungs and increases the risk of conditions such as chronic obstructive pulmonary disease (COPD) and pneumonia. It also worsens health conditions such as asthma and impacts fertility. Stopping smoking at any time has considerable health benefits. For more on smoking and health see the Action on Smoking (ASH) website at https://ash.org.uk/. Applying 'all our health' has more information on reducing harm from smoking in different populations groups who might present in healthcare settings. See more at https://www.gov.uk/government/publications/smoking-and-tobacco-applying-all-our-health/smoking-and-tobacco-applying-all-our-health.

Practitioner skills activity 5g: Supporting someone to stop smoking.
Have a look at this USA-based 'Smokefree' resource about helping someone to quit smoking at https://smokefree.gov/help-others-quit/how-to-support-someone-quitting. *Imagine you are helping Mohammed to stop smoking. He has been smoking for 20 years and wants to quit smoking as his wife is pregnant with their first child. What would you say to Mohammed about quitting smoking? What resources or support could you offer him?*

Stop smoking services are for people who want to quit smoking. They offer advice and support including one-to-one or small group support, or pharmacological aids such as Nicotine Replacement Therapy (NRT). Stop smoking support is also available online. In Canada, the Canadian government has 'tools for a smoke-free life' and has videos and resources to support quitters at https://www.canada.ca/en/health-canada/services/smoking-tobacco.html. It also has organisations that support those who want to stop. Smoke-Free Curious shows smokers what a smoke-free life might look like, for example, what more energy feels like and what freedom from cravings feels like. See more at https://www.smokefreecurious.ca/s/?language=en_US.

Health promotion in practice examples: Stopping smoking during pregnancy.
Babies born to mothers who smoke during pregnancy are more likely to be born early and be of lower birth weight. This can cause complications such as death and disability. In addition, adverse child outcomes from living in a smoking household include increased risk of respiratory infections and sudden infant death (SIDS). Guidance for health professionals in Australia suggests

that brief advice for pregnant women should be offered at every clinically appropriate opportunity in a clear, non-confrontational and personalised way. Read more at https://www.quitcentre.org.au/maternity. *A variety of free services exist to support pregnant women to be smoke-free. Hampshire (UK), has a 'Kickit' smoking in-pregnancy service which you can read more on here* https://www.smokefreehampshire.co.uk/smoking-in-pregnancy-kickit-campaign/. *SmokefreeMOM is a smoke-free text messaging service in the USA at* https://women.smokefree.gov/tools-tips-women/text-programs/smokefreemom.

In the UK stop smoking services are free to use and are delivered through a range of community health services. You can read about the UK stop smoking services for each NHS area; England Better Health at https://www.nhs.uk/better-health/quit-smoking/, Wales Health Help Me Quit at https://www.helpmequit.wales/, Quit your Way Scotland at https://www.nhsinform.scot/care-support-and-rights/nhs-services/helplines/quit-your-way-scotland, and Stop Smoking Northern Ireland at https://www.stopsmokingni.info/. Globally, many countries offer national stop-smoking quitlines. The WHO as part of their global quit kit has a list of quitlines and websites for many countries at https://www.who.int/campaigns/world-no-tobacco-day/2021/quitting-toolkit.

Health promotion in practice example: Florence the digital healthcare worker.

Florence is an Artificial Intelligence (A1) digital healthcare worker. She is the first WHO digital healthcare worker. She is designed to help people quit tobacco and e-cigarettes and to offer advice on stress, physical activity and nutrition. Meet Florence at https://www.who.int/campaigns/Florence.

COMMUNITY HEALTH WORKERS

Community health workers are healthcare providers who live in the communities in which they work and have some formal training or education but not at the same standard as health professionals in that country. They are most commonly used in low and middle-income countries to support the achievement of universal health coverage (UHC). Much of their remit is around the prevention of ill health and the management of disease in community-based settings. The

World Health Organization (2020) suggests that community health workers work in five main areas:

(1) **Delivering treatment, testing and/or clinical care:** For example screening services, blood pressure testing, distribution of contraceptives, and giving vaccinations.

(2) **Increasing uptake of health services and delivering health education:** For example giving knowledge, promoting the uptake of programmes and reducing stigma.

(3) **Being advocates or enablers between health systems and the community:** For example identifying community needs or challenges and reporting these to health centres.

(4) **Collecting data or record-keeping:** For example monitoring medication stocks or monitoring outbreaks.

(5) **Offering psychosocial support:** For example patient support groups or counselling.

An example of a community health worker scheme that covers all five of these areas is the Ethiopia community health extension programme that started in 2003. There are approximately 40,000 trained health extension workers in Ethiopia, and they form the 'community' part of Ethiopia's health system. They are attached to a small primary care unit and work with a health centre which serves approximately 25,000 people. Assefa et al. (2019) report that the programme has made significant achievements in maternal and child health, communicable disease, hygiene and sanitation, knowledge and health-seeking, and Rudgard et al. (2022) show improved adolescent health outcomes. Economic evaluations of the programme have also found interventions to be very cost-effective (Assebe et al., 2021) meaning they represent good value for money.

CLIMATE CHANGE-FRIENDLY HOSPITALS

Everyone in the world will experience the impacts of climate change, but those who are the most vulnerable will experience these impacts more than others. This includes the clinical or medically vulnerable. Hospitals are well-placed to be leaders in action against climate change. The NHS aims to become the world's first 'net-zero' emissions healthcare system. The 'Net Zero' plan (NHS England and NHS Health Improvement, 2020) outlines a target of net zero by 2040 for the emissions they directly control. This is known as the NHS 'Carbon Footprint'. The NHS is the biggest employer in the UK, and action needs to be taken to cut NHS emissions. The report identifies that around 4% of England's total carbon footprint is from the NHS. Solutions include immediate changes such as lighting and heating, but also adaptation and resilience strategies built into care. For more on climate change policy see Chapter 6 'Building healthy public policy'.

AIR POLLUTION AND CLIMATE-FRIENDLY HOSPITALS

SDG indicator 3.9 includes substantially reducing the number of deaths from air pollution. Many health benefits can be experienced by reducing fossil fuel emissions, as this will reduce air pollution. Reducing air pollution requires a health sector response and hospitals have the potential to reduce their emissions from a variety of sources. Figure 5.6 identifies some of these areas.

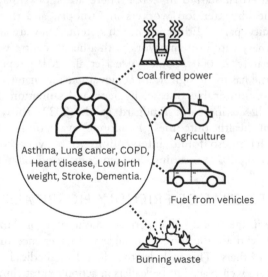

Figure 5.6 Hospitals and air pollution.

Poor air quality is one of the largest environmental risks to health globally. Reducing air pollution has substantial impacts on health, and these can rapidly be seen in areas where air pollution has been reduced by an immediate decrease in hospital admissions and all-cause mortality such as a cardiovascular and respiratory disease (Schraufnagel et al., 2019). Recent research suggests that air pollution impacts health negatively across the life course including pregnancy and birth outcomes such as low birth weight, child development including asthma and cognition, and adulthood such as chronic disease (Fuller et al., 2023). An easy-to-read explainer about air pollution is at the end of the chapter.

Reducing air pollution is a win–win situation for health. Additional health benefits can also be seen in solutions to reducing air pollution such as increasing physical activity levels through the promotion of safe, and active travel such as walking or bicycle paths. If we rely less on fossil fuels and more on renewable energy sources this can also cut energy costs in the long term. It also means less vulnerability to power shortages or the rising costs of fossil fuels. There are also potential savings in reduced hospital admissions and fewer premature deaths from poor air quality.

SEVEN AREAS OF A CLIMATE CHANGE-FRIENDLY HOSPITAL

The WHO and Healthcare Without Harm (2009) identify seven elements of a climate-friendly hospital in a discussion draft. Although this is an old document, the merits of this document lie in the holistic way it considers the hospitals of the future across the globe, as well as considering the major areas that healthy hospitals should focus on. The seven elements with examples are highlighted in Figure 5.7. They include energy efficiency, green building design, alternative energy generation, transportation, food, waste and water. Three of the seven areas are explained more below.

Practitioner skills activity 5h: Your local hospital.
Think about a hospital that you have visited or a hospital near where you live. Do you think it has acted in any of the seven areas? If you have been to your local hospital, what was the food like? Does it have outdoor spaces or

Energy efficiency: Switching to low energy lights, upgrading heating or cooling systems

Green building design: Using spaces for planting and growing, creating more natural spaces

Alternative energy: Using alternative power from solar, wind or biofuel

Transportation: Using electric vehicles, discounted public transport, promoting active travel

Food: Providing health meals, serving less meat, reducing food waste

Waste: Reducing, recycling, composting, reusing waste in all sectors

Water: Reducing water use through safe reuse and water conservation

Figure 5.7 Seven elements of a climate change-friendly hospital.

relaxation areas? How do you think it gets rid of its waste? Is it easy for people to get to the hospital using public transport?

GREEN BUILDING DESIGN

Newly built hospitals should consider climate change in building design and construction. This might be using current spaces for planting, food growing and creating green or natural spaces within the hospital spaces and grounds. Ideas like green roofs (plants on a roof) and living walls (usually plants growing vertically in soil or water–based nutrients) can have major environmental benefit for wildlife and offers insulation and temperature control benefits.

TRANSPORTATION

Hospitals usually have a 'fleet' of vehicles. This includes ambulances and delivery vehicles that bring supplies to the hospital like medicines as well as staff and patient transport. Alternative fuel vehicles such as electric vehicles or bio-diesel fuels, discounted bus transport, car sharing, or safe bicycle routes can reduce transportation.

WASTE

Hospitals have a lot of waste. Reducing waste through recycling, composting, procuring projects with less packaging, and buying reusable products can all reduce waste. Recycling facilities and schemes such as reusing cups or water bottles can also reduce waste for hospital staff and visitors.

REORIENTATING HEALTH PROMOTION RESEARCH

One of the challenges in health promotion is finding evidence for action. There is often plenty of evidence for the problem, for example, air pollution causing poor respiratory health (see previous section on air pollution). What is less clear are the solutions to preventing or reducing the problem. This is often because interventions that focus on prevention, for example preventing air pollution, are influenced by multiple factors at the individual, community and environmental levels. Some of this research must therefore come from areas outside of health, such as transport and industry that, in part, cause the problem.

Practitioner skills activity 5i: Finding evidence for the prevention of ischaemic heart disease.

Imagine you want to plan a health promotion initiative that reduces people's risk of heart disease. Where would you get evidence-based interventions to help you decide on what to do? If you wanted to address some of the wider determinants of health that might increase people's risks of heart disease, where would you find this information?

Health promotion evidence that is available is often skewed (meaning biased) to Randomised Control Trials (RCTs). RCTs are considered to be one of the best types of evidence available for proof of effectiveness. They are conducted in a carefully controlled environment and are often used in medicine. There are fewer RCTs in health promotion. This is because many factors influence the outcome of an intervention or campaign and these are very difficult to control. For example, an intervention to reduce loneliness in older people could be influenced by their age, their retirement status, where they live, their disposable income, their friendships and so on. This makes it difficult to design RCTs in health promotion as we can't carefully control people.

Most research that is conducted in health promotion focuses on changing individual behaviours (see Chapter 2 'Developing personal skills'), rather than policy environments or whole settings (see Chapter 6 'Building healthy public policy' and Chapter 4 'Creating supportive environments'). This means it is much more common to find individual behaviour change interventions and much less easy to evidence at the policy or environmental level.

EVIDENCE IN HEALTH PROMOTION

When we work in health promotion practice, where possible we need to use evidence to support what we do. Using the best available evidence for our action justifies that what we are doing is safe, effective and appropriate and it is likely to help us achieve what we set out to do. There are numerous places where we can obtain evidence for health promotion action. If you attend a university and study a health subject, you will be taught how to use 'library databases'. These are large databases of journals which publish articles on different topics relevant to health. Some journal articles can be accessed without a subscription. For example, the National Library of Medicine hosts 'PubMed' which can be used without a subscription to locate information, although not all the articles are free. See more at https://pubmed.ncbi.nlm.nih.gov/.

Cochrane reviews are different types of systematic reviews of health evidence. A systematic review is like a summary of all the quality research in a specific area. These reviews are relevant across a wide range of areas, for example, the most recent reviews at the time of writing include listening to music to prevent insomnia (Jespersen et al., 2022), smoking cessation for secondary prevention of cardiovascular disease (Wu et al., 2022) and replacing salt with low-sodium substitutes for cardiovascular health (Brand et al., 2022). You can find more evidence at https://www.cochranelibrary.com/.

Globally, large organisations have useful resources for health promotion evidence. For example, the United Nations SDG website has a wide range of publications for ways to implement the SDGs at https://sdgs.un.org/publications. In the UK organisations like the Health Foundation https://www.health.org.uk/ or The King's Fund https://www.kingsfund.org.uk/ offer a wide range of reports, policy documents and evidence for action. The National Institute of Health and Care Excellence (NICE) provides evidence-based guidance across a whole range of settings. This includes guidance and standards around core areas such as settings, lifestyle and well-being, health protection and population groups. Two examples from the NICE website are: Improving the environment to support physical activity https://www.nice.org.uk/guidance/ng90 and mental well-being at work https://www.nice.org.uk/guidance/ng90.

Health promotion in practice example: WHO-CHOICE and cost-effectiveness evidence.

The World Health Organization (2021c) tool for choosing cost-effective interventions (WHO-CHOICE) publishes evidence that shows interventions that are cost-effective in low-income settings. There is a downloadable tool for countries to create cost estimates. It gives examples of interventions in areas such as maternal health, non-communicable diseases, HIV, TB and malaria and universal health coverage (UHC). For example, for maternal and child health high-value interventions include family planning, neonatal resuscitation, Vitamin A, measles vaccines, and management of neonatal infection. See more at https://www.ijhpm.com/issue_694_705.html.

EVALUATING HEALTH PROMOTION

One area of health promotion that needs more attention is evaluation. This is partly because practitioners who deliver health promotion do not always have formal training, and also because evaluation can be difficult to do. The examples in the evidence section explained how evidence can be difficult to find, and this is often because campaigns and projects are not well evaluated.

Evaluation helps us to see what works well, and what does not work as well as several other useful measures, for example, how many people attended each week? How much money was spent? Or what do the participants think about the intervention? Evaluation always measures the original aim or objectives of the health promotion campaign or intervention. For example, an increase in knowledge or the development of a skill.

There are four main broad categories of evaluation. These are shown in Figure 5.8.

The four evaluation areas in Figure 5.8 are:

PROCESS EVALUATION

This is measuring the process of the intervention such as testing that the campaign materials are suitable or that the training went as planned. For example, did your radio message get announced correctly? Or where were your media messages seen?

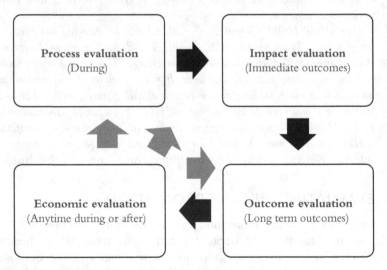

Figure 5.8 Evaluation in health promotion.

IMPACT EVALUATION

This is the immediate impact of the intervention, such as how many people can show a skill or recall knowledge after a workshop or activity. For example, can participants show you five exercises? Or can someone teach back to you what you told them about their medication?

OUTCOME EVALUATION

This is the long-term impact of the intervention, including how many people are still doing the behaviour or activity. For example, how many people are smoke-free at three months? Or how many people are still eating a lower-sodium diet at six months?

ECONOMIC EVALUATION

This is an evaluation linked to the cost of a programme. Most commonly economic evaluations are used to see if an intervention is cost-effective, or cost-saving. Cost-effective means that the money spent was less than reasonable alternatives or to a specific amount of money. Cost-saving is the amount of money saved, usually in the long term or compared to alternatives. In health promotion, the amount of money is frequently calculated from a healthcare perspective. 'Money saved' is calculated in terms of mortality such as how many life years are saved, or morbidity, such as life years lived without a disability. There can be wider societal costs saved as well, for example a programme that helps people manage their chronic disease could calculate the days of work where someone is not absent for a health-related illness. A programme that aims to reduce truancy or school exclusion in high-risk young people could look at money saved from criminal justice systems. For more on economic evaluation see the resources at the end of the chapter, and the WHO-CHOICE tool in the health promotion in practice example above.

Practitioner skills activity 5j: Evaluating a breastfeeding promotion intervention.

You want to deliver a health promotion intervention in a local community. This will be supported by two health visitors and will encourage mothers to breastfeed for at least six months. Your intervention will use social media and face-to-face support through health visitors and peers (mother to mother). What could you evaluate in the process evaluation? Impact evaluation? And outcome evaluation? Try and think of at least two questions for each.

There are several resources to support health promoters in evaluation. Interventions that aim to change behaviour or knowledge often make use of pre and post-tests (often questionnaires) to ask what people know or do before an intervention, and what people know or do after an intervention, to see if there is a change. Several freely available validated tools can be used for this purpose in hundreds of different topic areas. For example, an intervention that aims to increase health literacy might evaluate health literacy before and after an intervention, and measure this with a health literacy tool. Examples of tools to measure health literacy can be found here https://healthliteracy.bu.edu/. For brief interventions, the Royal Society of Public Health provides Impact pathways for everyday healthcare interactions to help practitioners measure the work they do with people. This resource can be found at https://www.rsph.org.uk/our-work/policy/wider-public-health-workforce/measuring-public-health-impact.html.

SUMMARY

Everyone who works in health has a responsibility to change. Every health service has the potential to be better. Every organisation has the power to transform. If we don't change, we will continue to exclude those who need our care the most and we will continue to prioritise cure over prevention. This is unsustainable and costly both financially and for people's health. Health promoters have much potential to offer their expertise and guidance in reorientating healthcare services to prevention, as well as providing evidence and evaluating current work to showcase the potential of what can be done to move from 'cure' to 'prevention'.

Many changes to healthcare services can be supported through the building of healthy public policy, and stronger health policies will also mean less need for costly healthcare. The final chapter of the book, therefore, moves to building 'Healthy public policy'.

WIDER READING

ONLINE

UK Government (2022). NHS Migrant health guide. Available at https://www.gov.uk/guidance/nhs-entitlements-migrant-health-guide.

Action for clean air has a clean air hospital framework resource at https://www.actionforcleanair.org.uk/health/clean-air-hospital-framework and resources for schools and businesses at https://www.actionforcleanair.org.uk/.

Public Health England (2018). Health matters: Air pollution. https://www.gov.uk/government/publications/health-matters-air-pollution/health-matters-air-pollution.

Buck, D., & Ewbank, L. (2020). What is social prescribing. https://www.kingsfund.org.uk/publications/social-prescribing.

BITC/Public Health England (2019). Health and well-being toolkits. https://www.bitc.org.uk/toolkit/take-a-whole-system-approach-to-health/.

For more on health economics and cost-effectiveness have a look at Public Health England (2021). Health economics: A Guide for public health teams at https://www.gov.uk/guidance/health-economics-a-guide-for-public-health-teams.

TEXTBOOKS

Hollnager, E., Braithwaite, J., & Wears, R. L. (2018). *Delivering resilient healthcare*. Routledge, London.

McCormack, D., McCance, T., Bulley, C., Brown, D., McMillan, A., & Martin, S. (2021). *Fundamentals of person-centred healthcare practice*. John Wiley & Sons, Oxford.

LISTENING AND WATCHING

The King's Fund podcasts: 'Supporting Refugee and Migrant Health in England' and 'Leading with Compassion. Supporting the health and well-being of healthcare staff' is available from The King's Fund website https://www.kingsfund.org.uk/ or your podcast provider.

ADDITIONAL REFERENCES

These are the additional references this chapter has used where electronic links have not been provided in the chapter.

Assebe, L. F., Belete, W. N., Alemayehu, S., Asfaw, E., Godana, K. T., Alemayehu, Y. K., Teklu, A. M., & Yigezu, A. (2021). Economic evaluation of health extension program packages in Ethiopia. *PLoS One*, *16*(2), e0246207. 10.1371/journal.pone.0246207.

Assefa, Y., Gelaw, Y. A., Hill, P. S., Taye, B. W., & Van Damme, W. (2019). Community health extension program of Ethiopia, 2003-2018: Successes and challenges toward universal coverage for primary healthcare services. *Global Health*, *15*(1), 24. 10.1186/s12992-019-0470-1.

Ayele, A. A., Cosh, S., Islam, M. S., & East, L. (2022). Role of community pharmacy professionals in child health service provision in Ethiopia: A cross-sectional survey in six cities of Amhara regional state. *BMC Health Services Research*, *22*(1), 1259. 10.1186/s12913-022-08641-8.

Brand, A., Visser, M. E., Schoonees, A., & Naude, C. E. (2022). Replacing salt with low-sodium salt substitutes (LSSS) for cardiovascular health in adults, children and pregnant women. *Cochrane Database of Systematic Reviews*, (8). 10.1002/14651858.CD015207.

Bristol, S., Kostelec, T., & MacDonald, R. (2018). Improving emergency health care workers' knowledge, competency, and attitudes toward lesbian, gay, bisexual, and transgender patients through interdisciplinary cultural competency training. *Journal of Emergency Nursing*, *44*(6), 632–639. 10.1016/j.jen.2018.03.013.

Cream, J., Fenny, D., Williams, E., Baylis, A., Dahir, S., & Wyatt, H. (2020). Delivering health and care for people who sleep rough: Going above and beyond. Available at https://www.kingsfund.org.uk/publications/delivering-health-care-people-sleep-rough.

Crisis UK. (2022). *Homelessness knowledge hub*. Available at https://www.crisis.org.uk/ending-homelessness/homelessness-knowledge-hub/.

Curtis, E., Jones, R., Tipene-Leach, D., Walker, C., Loring, B., Paine, S. J., & Reid, P. (2019). Why cultural safety rather than cultural competency is required to achieve health equity: A literature review and recommended definition. *International Journal Equity Health*, *18*(1), 174. 10.1186/s12939-019-1082-3.

Department of Health and Social Care. (2019). UK 20-year vision for anti-microbial resistance. Available at https://www.gov.uk/government/collections/antimicrobial-resistance-amr-information-and-resources.

Department of Health and Social Care. (2021). Good for you, good for us, good for everybody: A plan to reduce overprescribing to make patient care better and safer, support the NHS, and reduce carbon emissions. Available at https://www.gov.uk/government/publications/national-overprescribing-review-report.

Fair, F., Raben, L., Watson, H., Vivilaki, V., van den Muijsenbergh, M., & Soltani, H. (2020). Migrant women's experiences of pregnancy, childbirth and maternity care in European countries: A systematic review. *PLoS One*, *15*(2), e0228378. 10.1371/journal.pone.0228378.

Fuller, G., Friedman, S., Mudway, I., Environmental Research Group., & London., I. C. (2023). Impacts of air pollution across the life course – Evidence highlight note. Available at https://www.london.gov.uk/sites/default/files/2023-04/Imperial%20College%20London%20Projects%20-%20impacts%20of%20air%20pollution%20across%20the%20life%20course%20%E2%80%93%20evidence%20highlight%20note.pdf.

Government Equalities Office. (2010). Equality Act 2010: Guidance. Available at https://www.gov.uk/guidance/equality-act-2010-guidance.

Groundswell and Crisis. (2021). #HealthNow peer research report: Understanding homeless health inequality in Birmingham. Available at https://www.crisis.org.uk/ending-homelessness/homelessness-knowledge-hub/health-and-wellbeing/healthnow-peer-research-report-understanding-homeless-health-inequality-in-birmingham-2021/.

Jespersen, K. V., Pando-Naude, V., Koenig, J., Jennum, P., & Vuust, P. (2022). Listening to music for insomnia in adults. *Cochrane Database of Systematic Reviews*, (8). 10.1002/14651858.CD010459.pub3.

Kearns, R. A., Neuwelt, P. M., & Eggleton, K. (2020). Permeable boundaries? Patient perspectives on space and time in general practice waiting rooms. *Health & Place*, *63*, 102347. 10.1016/j.healthplace.2020.102347.

Kneck, Å., Klarare, A., Mattsson, E., & Salzmann-Erikson, M. (2022). Reflections on health among women in homelessness: A qualitative study. *J Psychiatr Ment Health Nurs*, *29*(5), 709–720. 10.1111/jpm.12859.

Luchenski, S., Maguire, N., Aldridge, R. W., Hayward, A., Story, A., Perri, P., Withers, J., Clint, S., Fitzpatrick, S., & Hewett, N. (2018). What works in inclusion health: Overview of effective interventions for marginalised and excluded populations. *Lancet*, *391*(10117), 266–280. 10.1016/s0140-6736(17)31959-1.

Melo, A. C., Trindade, G. M., Freitas, A. R., Resende, K. A., & Palhano, T. J. (2021). Community pharmacies and pharmacists in Brazil: A missed opportunity. *Pharm Pract (Granada)*, *19*(2), 2467. 10.18549/PharmPract.2021.2.2467.

Mosites, E., Hughes, L., & Butler, J. C. (2022). Homelessness and infectious diseases: Understanding the gaps and defining a public health approach. *The Journal of Infectious Diseases*, *226*(Supplement_3), S301–S303. 10.1093/infdis/jiac352.

National Institute for Clinical Excellence. (2015). Antimicrobial stewardship: Systems and processes for effective antimicrobial medicine use NICE guideline [NG15]. Available at https://www.nice.org.uk/guidance/ng15.

NHS. (2019). The NHS longterm plan. Available at https://www.longtermplan.nhs.uk/publication/nhs-long-term-plan/.

NHS England and NHS Health Improvement (2020). Delivering a Net Zero National Health Service. Available at https://www.england.nhs.uk/greenernhs/wp-content/uploads/sites/51/2020/10/delivering-a-net-zero-national-health-service.pdf.

NHS Inform (Scotland). (2021). Chronic pain self-help guide. Available at https://www.nhsinform.scot/illnesses-and-conditions/mental-health/mental-health-self-help-guides/chronic-pain-self-help-guide.

O'Mahony, D., O'Sullivan, D., Byrne, S., O'Connor, M. N., Ryan, C., & Gallagher, P. (2015). STOPP/START criteria for potentially inappropriate prescribing in older people: version 2. *Age Ageing*, *44*(2), 213–218. 10.1093/ageing/afu145.

Office for Health Improvement and Disparities. (2022). Community centred practice: Applying all our health. Available at https://www.gov.uk/government/publications/community-centred-practice-applying-all-our-health.

Office of National Statistics. (2021a). Deaths of homeless people in England and Wales: 2020 registrations. Available at https://www.ons.gov.uk/peoplepopulationandcommunity/birthsdeathsandmarriages/deaths/bulletins/deathsofhomelesspeopleinenglandandwales/2020registrations.

Office of National Statistics. (2021b). National life tables – life expectancy in the UK: 2018 to 2020. Available at https://www.ons.gov.uk/peoplepopulationandcommunity/birthsdeathsandmarriages/lifeexpectancies/bulletins/nationallifetablesunitedkingdom/2018to2020.

Papps, E., & Ramsden, I. (1996). Cultural safety in nursing: The New Zealand experience. *Int J Qual Health Care*, *8*(5), 491–497. 10.1093/intqhc/8.5.491.

Pinheiro, M. B., Sherrington, C., Howard, K., Caldwell, P., Tiedemann, A., Wang, B., J, S. O., Santos, A., Bull, F. C., Willumsen, J. F., Michaleff, Z. A., Ferguson, S., Mayo, E., Fairhall, N. J., Bauman, A. E., & Norris, S. (2022). Economic evaluations of fall prevention exercise programs: A systematic review. *Br J Sports Med*, *56*(23), 1353–1365. 10.1136/bjsports-2022-105747.

Public Health England. (2017). Health and wellbeing in rural areas. Available at https://www.local.gov.uk/sites/default/files/documents/1.39_Health%20in%20rural%20areas_WEB.pdf.

Public Health England. (2019a). Guidance about 'All our Health'. Available at https://www.gov.uk/government/publications/all-our-health-about-the-framework/all-our-health-about-the-framework.

Public Health England. (2019b). Health matters: Stopping smoking – What works? Available at https://www.gov.uk/government/publications/health-matters-stopping-smoking-what-works/health-matters-stopping-smoking-what-works.

Rudgard, W. E., Dzumbunu, S. P., Yates, R., Toska, E., Stöckl, H., Hertzog, L., Emaway, D., & Cluver, L. (2022). Multiple impacts of ethiopia's health extension program on adolescent health and well-being: A quasi-experimental study 2002–2013. *Journal of Adolescent Health*, *71*(3), 308–316. 10.1016/j.jadohealth.2022.04.010.

Schraufnagel, D. E., Balmes, J. R., De Matteis, S., Hoffman, B., Kim, W. J., Perez-Padilla, R., Rice, M., Sood, A., Vanker, A., & Wuebbles, D. J. (2019).

Health benefits of air pollution reduction. *Annals of American Thoracic Society*, *16*(12), 1478–1487. 10.1513/AnnalsATS.201907-538CME.

Stonewall UK. (2023). UK workplace equality index. Available at https://www.stonewall.org.uk/creating-inclusive-workplaces/workplace-equality-indices/uk-workplace-equality-index.

The Health Foundation. (2019). The NHS as an anchor institution. Available at https://www.health.org.uk/news-and-comment/charts-and-infographics/the-nhs-as-an-anchor-institution.

Thomson, K., Hillier-Brown, F., Walton, N., Bilaj, M., Bambra, C., & Todd, A. (2019). The effects of community pharmacy-delivered public health interventions on population health and health inequalities: A review of reviews. *Preventive Medicine*, *124*, 98–109. 10.1016/j.ypmed.2019.04.003.

Torjesen, I. (2016). Social prescribing could help alleviate pressure on GPs. *BMJ*, *352*, i1436. 10.1136/bmj.i1436.

Urbanoski, K., Pauly, B., Inglis, D., Cameron, F., Haddad, T., Phillips, J., Phillips, P., Rosen, C., Schlotter, G., Hartney, E., & Wallace, B. (2020). Defining culturally safe primary care for people who use substances: A participatory concept mapping study. *BMC Health Serv Res*, *20*(1), 1060. 10.1186/s12913-020-05915-x.

World Health Organization. (2020). What do we know about community health workers? A systematic review of existing reviews. Available at https://apps.who.int/iris/handle/10665/340717.

World Health Organization. (2021a). Falls. Available at https://www.who.int/news-room/fact-sheets/detail/falls.

World Health Organization. (2021b). Step safely: Strategies for preventing and managing falls across the life-course. Available at https://www.who.int/teams/social-determinants-of-health/safety-and-mobility/step-safely.

World Health Organization. (2021c). WHO choice tool new updates. Available at https://www.who.int/news-room/feature-stories/detail/new-cost-effectiveness-updates-from-who-choice.

World Health Organization. (2022). Tobacco. Available at https://www.who.int/news-room/fact-sheets/detail/tobacco

World Health Organization and Healthcare without Harm. (2009). Healthy Hospitals, healthy planet, healthy people. Available at https://www.who.int/docs/default-source/climate-change/healthy-hospitals-healthy-planet-healthy-people.pdf?sfvrsn=8b337cee_1.

Wu, A. D., Lindson, N., Hartmann-Boyce, J., Wahedi, A., Hajizadeh, A., Theodoulou, A., Thomas, E. T., Lee, C., & Aveyard, P. (2022). Smoking cessation for secondary prevention of cardiovascular disease. *Cochrane Database of Systematic Reviews*, (8). 10.1002/14651858.CD014936.pub2.

BUILDING HEALTHY PUBLIC POLICY

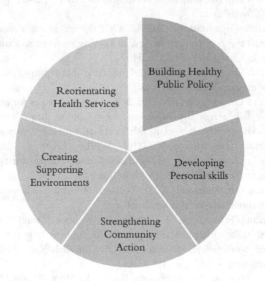

Figure 6.1 Building health public policy.

DOI: 10.4324/9781003462323-7

- Five things health promoters might do to build healthy public policy
- Overview
- What is a healthy public policy?
- Transport policies and health
- Country health policies
- Using Government law for health and well-being
- Benchmarking
- Good governance
- Universal health coverage (UHC)
- The health promoter's role in policy making
- Policy consultation process
- Making a healthy policy
- Identifying the problem and solution generation
- Decision making
- Implementation and evaluation
- Health Impact Assessments (HIAs)
- Different policies for different purposes
- The intervention ladder
- Tackling illegal drugs through policies
- Tackling climate change through policies
- Promoting active travel through policies
- Reducing adolescent pregnancy through policies
- Challenges to healthy public policy
- Summary
- Wider reading

FIVE THINGS HEALTH PROMOTERS MIGHT DO TO BUILD HEALTHY PUBLIC POLICY

(1) Attending consultations to give feedback on proposed Government policies that impact health.
(2) Coordinating stakeholders and writing a group response when Governments ask for feedback or evidence on proposed policies.
(3) Holding community workshops to gather evidence about the health priorities and needs of communities.

(4)   Making connections to non-health sector organisations to ensure their policies prioritise health.

(5)   Benchmarking what other countries or organisations are doing to promote health and using ideas to make policy better (Figure 6.1).

OVERVIEW

A policy is a law, guidance or plan of action that tries to shape or change something. Policies are in place to support the way we live. It would be very difficult to live in a place without any. For example, people who work will have laws and policies which tell them about their job responsibilities, how their employer will keep them safe and what actions are in place to protect them in their job. If these policies didn't exist workers might not know what they are supposed to do in their job or how to do their job safely. This provides some of the rationale for SDG 8 'decent work and economic growth' that focuses on creating safe and secure working environments for all. A global example is that of readymade garment workers in some South Asian countries. Have a look at the clothes that you are wearing. Do you know where your clothes were made? Some clothes are made in factories where working conditions are poor. Garment workers experience a wide range of risks to their health through unsafe and hazardous working environments where there are very few laws in place to protect them (Kabir et al., 2019). You can read more about garment workers and about the campaign to improve responsibility in UK clothing at https://www.waronwant.org/our-work/garment-workers.

The word policy can be interpreted differently depending on who is using the word. Similar words like 'Law', 'Legislation', 'and 'Act' may be used.

- A law is a formal act published by a legislative body, like the Government, and applies to everyone. An 'Act' of parliament is a 'Law'.
- A 'Policy' is made by groups of people in charge of something like a local council and may only apply to certain people.

An example of a formal 'Law' or 'Act' is that tobacco smoking is not allowed in enclosed workplaces, public buildings or on public transport in the UK (UK Government, 2022). Those who do not comply can be fined. Policies are what organisations use, for example, a school, workplace or local council. They might tell you what to do each day, or outline how to keep people safe from harm. 'Healthy Public policy' includes both laws and policies.

WHAT IS A HEALTHY PUBLIC POLICY?

A healthy public policy shows concern for health and equity in all areas of policy. It is accountable (meaning responsible) for the impact of what it says on health (World Health Organization, 1986). It should improve the conditions in which people live. This could be through policies that support good quality housing, the provision of clean water or community services. Improving and protecting health can be done in different ways. For example, to reduce emissions from air pollution we would need to look at the different sectors that are polluting the air and create policies in these areas. Here are four examples of sources of air pollution where we could look at building healthy public policies.

- Transport, through petrol and diesel vehicles.
- Homes, though burning wood and coal for heating or cooking.
- Farming, through adding fertilizer or other farming methods.
- Industry, through making foods or products like clothes.

TRANSPORT POLICIES AND HEALTH

Many policies are made by different sectors outside of healthcare. Policies to reduce road traffic accidents, increase safety and regulation of transport and manage transport demand are important in improving transport safety. This includes separating traffic (vehicles, cycles and pedestrians), improving the conditions of roads and road user regulations such as speeding measures. Figure 6.2 shows an example of road transport policies. It includes the macro (or wider) environment and the micro (community) environment. These are explained below.

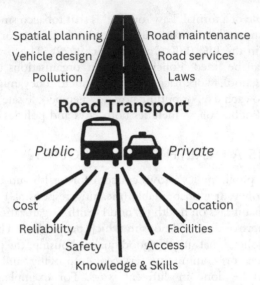

Figure 6.2 Road transport policies.

Macro policies include:

- Spatial planning. These influence the need to use transport it dictates where shops or houses will be built.
- Laws around road safety, provision of roadside services and vehicle design. These influence health by preventing (or not) road traffic accidents.
- Air pollution from transport. This contributes to higher morbidity and mortality rates.

Micro policies include:

- Policies around cost, reliability, safety, access and the provision of facilities in transport hubs like bus stations. These impact on people's experiences and choices when using transport.
- Individual knowledge and skills. These are needed to legally drive vehicles or navigate public transport such as the provisions of timetables.

To improve health through transport, for example, by increasing the number of people who use public transport instead of private vehicles thus reducing pollution, we would need to look at the macro and the micro policy environment. Transport is a complex issue and it requires both those from the health sector and those from the transport sector to work together. See the health promotion in practice example below about road safety in China.

Health promotion in practice example: Active travel and road safety challenges in China.

There are numerous challenges associated with promoting active travel and road safety in China. Research by Jiang et al. (2017) states that education is not the way to promote road safety. They report that education programmes alone will not have an impact on road safety if the road conditions are not improved, and adequate incentives are not in place to obey traffic laws. They also note that one of the difficulties is that transport and health are often looked at as two separate issues. For example, actioning active travel is limited by transport infrastructures and air pollution. Those choosing active travel are at risk of outdoor air pollution, risks in road environments, and risk through insufficient medical services in case of an accident. This means changes are needed in different sectors and across different levels for the health benefits of active travel to be seen.

Some policies have multiple benefits, for example, low emission zones in cities such as London's (England) Ultra Low Emission Zone mean vehicles have to comply with emission zone laws or pay a fee to drive in that area. This policy reduces congestion, reduces air pollution and reduces climate change. Read more at https://tfl. gov.uk/modes/driving/ultra-low-emission-zone. A useful resource for an international perspective on how policy impacts health is 'The Lancet Voice' podcast https://www.thelancet.com/podcasts.

COUNTRY HEALTH POLICIES

Many countries have health policies which outline priority areas for action. The most well-known global targets are the Sustainable Development Goals (SDGs) which specify actions for all countries across 17 goals. See Chapter 1 for more on the SDGs. Many countries also have a public health or health promotion national policy. Below are examples from the four countries that make up the UK.

England has a 2020–2025 'Public health strategy' document with 10 priorities including a smoke-free society, healthier diets healthier weight, cleaner air and better mental health. Read more at Public Health England (2019) https://www.gov.uk/government/publications/phe-strategy-2020-to-2025.

Wales outlines priorities in a long-term strategy for 2018–2030 called 'Working to achieve a healthier future for Wales'. Priorities include influencing the wider determinants of health, improving mental well-being and promoting healthy behaviours. Read more at Public Health Wales (2018) https://phw.nhs.wales/about-us/our-priorities/.

In Scotland, there are six public health priorities including 'A Scotland where we live in vibrant, healthy and safe places and communities' and 'A Scotland where we reduce the use of and harm from alcohol, tobacco and other drugs'. Read more at Scottish Government (2018) https://www.gov.scot/publications/scotlands-public-health-priorities/documents/.

Northern Ireland uses a whole system framework titled 'Making life better' for 2013–2023. It includes six themes such as 'giving every child the best start' and 'empowering healthy living'. Read more at Department of Health (2014) (NI) https://www.health-ni.gov.uk/articles/making-life-better-strategic-framework-public-health.

Practitioner skills activity 2a: If you were in charge …

If you were in charge of creating a health policy for the country in which you live, which five areas would you choose as your priorities? Why would you choose these areas? What did you base your decision-making on? Do you think there is good evidence for ways to address your chosen priorities?

USING GOVERNMENT LAW FOR HEALTH AND WELL-BEING

Some countries use Government laws to prioritise health and well-being. For example, Wales has a 'Well-being of Future Generations (Wales) Act (Welsh Government, 2015) discussed in the example below. New Zealand has a budget specifically focused on health and well-being. In 2022 this was adapted to include culturally appropriate well-being frameworks. Read more at New Zealand Government (2022) https://budget.govt.nz/budget/2022/wellbeing/outlook/index.htm. The Well-being Economy Alliance contains videos and resources about the well-being economy Government commitments from Finland, Iceland, New Zealand, Scotland and Wales at https:// weall.org/.

Health promotion in practice example: The Well-being of Future Generations (Wales) Act.

The Well-being of Future Generations (Wales) Act (2015) requires all policymakers to commit to prioritizing well-being. This means thinking of the long-term health impacts of the planned policy, regardless of the policy area. The act has seven well-being goals that contribute to the social, economic, environmental and cultural well-being of Wales. These are: A prosperous Wales, A resilient Wales, A healthier Wales, A more equal Wales, A Wales of cohesive communities, A Wales of vibrant culture and thriving Welsh language, and A globally responsible Wales. These are shown in Figure 6.3. The Act is underpinned by sustainable development principles, and all local authorities produce an area well-being plan. Progress is measured through well-being goals. Read more at https://gov.wales/ well-being-future-generations *or watch the short animation at* https:// www.youtube.com/watch?v=rFeOYlxJbmw.

BENCHMARKING

Benchmarking is a way of comparing progress in an organisation, region or country with progress in another comparable location. As an example, we might look at the average percentage of pupils who are absent from school across a country, and then schools would measure their percentages and benchmark these against their levels. We might then look at which schools are doing well reducing pupil absence and explore what solutions we could replicate in other schools.

Benchmarking helps regions like councils or authorities and large organisations to measure progress and look at areas that need more work. One difficulty in benchmarking is what is used as a comparison. The countries, regions, or organisations that are benchmarked against the need to be similar or share some common features. Countries have different geographies and populations as well as their own cultural, social, political, economic and health systems and structures. What works in one place may not work in another place.

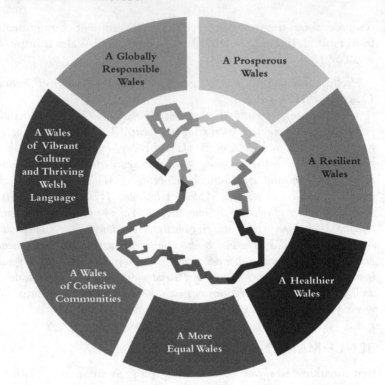

Figure 6.3 The Well-being of Future Generations (Wales) Act (2015).

Health promotion in practice example: Health promotion benchmarking in Finland.

In Finland, municipalities are responsible for promoting the health of people who live in those areas. TEAViisari is a tool developed to promote policies informed by evidence. The tool shows actions that different municipalities take and provides information on that action. It measures areas like how organisations are committed to health promotion, the resources that are in place for health promotion and how health needs are monitored. See the tool at https://teaviisari.fi/teaviisari/en/index?

Tools are available to help policymakers benchmark against other countries. The European Social Progress Index (EU–SPI) (European Commission, 2023) aims to measure social progress for each EU region as a complement to traditional measures of economic progress, such as the Gross Domestic Product (GDP). GDP is a measure of how much an economy is growing. The EU-SPI measures 12 components across three broad areas shown below:

- **Basic human needs:** These include nutrition and basic medical care, shelter, water and sanitation and personal security.
- **Foundations of well-being:** These include access to basic knowledge, access to information and communication, health and wellness, and environmental quality.
- **Opportunity:** This includes personal rights, personal freedom of choice, tolerance and inclusion, and access to advanced education.

The EU-SPI allows regions to see their scores compared to other regions and different countries. All top-ten regions are in Sweden, Finland or Denmark. See the activity below to learn more about the EU-SPI.

Practitioner skills activity 2b: Benchmarking EU countries using the EU-SPI.

Look at the 2020 EE-SPI results and explore the maps or scorecards between EU countries. The online data story can help you navigate through the results and shows you the key points at https://cohesiondata.ec.europa.eu/stories/s/EU-Social-Progress-Index-2020/8qk9-xq96.

GOOD GOVERNANCE

Good governance is about making sure that those people who make policies are responsible for their actions and decisions. SDG 16 is focused on 'peaceful, inclusive societies for sustainable development' which includes developing effective, accountable and transparent institutions. This means people who are in charge and make decisions about public services must ensure they are safe and well-managed as well as protecting stakeholders involved in service delivery. Governance is a process where the organisations delivering services, policies or programmes have to deliver the right services in the right way. Delivery is monitored against clearly stated outcomes or measures.

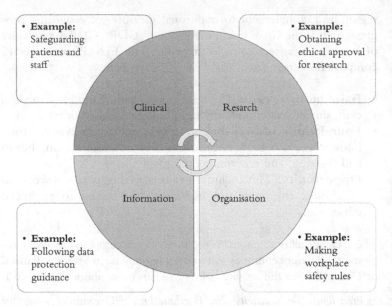

Figure 6.4 Different types of governance.

There are different types of governance including clinical governance, research governance, organisation governance and information governance.

Figure 6.4. shows examples of the different types of governance.

- **Clinical governance** refers to health sector accountability such as improving standards of care, managing risks and safeguarding patients and resources.
- **Research governance** is connected to the regulations and standards for good quality research.
- **Organisation governance** is important for how organisations work and how resources and people are managed.
- **Information governance** includes data protection and security of systems that collect data.

Health promoters can advocate for sectors to be more accountable for the health effects of their products. This is called 'corporate responsibility'. It means organisations have to put measures into place to protect people from the harm their products might cause. The Global Alliance on Breastfeeding states that countries should 'adopt and monitor the 'International code of marketing of breastmilk substitutes'; see https://www.globalbreastfeedingcollective.org/. The Lancet series on breast-feeding for example draws attention to the way the commercial milk formula industry uses aggressive marketing techniques and Government lobbying to promote their products. In 1981 the World Health Assembly adopted a set of standards to prevent the inappropriate marketing of formula, including banning free samples but only 32 countries have legal policies in place that strongly reflect the code. Read more at https://www.thelancet.com/series/Breastfeeding-2023.

Progress has been better in other areas, for example, tobacco companies in many countries now tell people that tobacco damages health on tobacco packets and many countries now only sell cigarettes in plain packets. However, progress still needs improvement. For example in the EU, young people and women remain the frequent targets of tobacco advertising, promotion or sponsorship, and many countries have only banned direct mass media advertising, not indirect advertising or other forms of direct advertising (World Health Organization, 2023). The example below shows suggestions for improving virtual environments.

Health promotion in practice example: The internet, suicide and self-harm (UK).

The internet and social media can be used to search for content on how people can hurt themselves (self-harm or suicide). There are very few restrictions that protect people from being able to do this. The Samaritans (2023) are campaigning for all internet sites and social media platforms to take an active role in reducing access to harmful content. Suggestions for what organisations can do include developing safety functions so users can block content, prioritising self-harm support services in search results, and adding sensitivity content warnings. An online safety bill is currently being debated in UK Parliament to make online content safer. You can see the progress of this bill at https://bills.parliament.uk/bills/3137.

UNIVERSAL HEALTH COVERAGE (UHC)

Healthcare is not free. It has to be paid for in some way, usually partly through the Government and partly through collecting taxes or paying money into an insurance scheme. Not all countries have well-funded healthcare systems. Universal Health Coverage (UHC) is when people have access to good quality health services without experiencing financial problems to get this care. It covers all the essential health services that support the prevention of ill health and the treatment of disease. SDG 3 'good health and well-being' includes indicator 3.8 which is to 'achieve universal health coverage including access to essential healthcare services, and safe, effective, quality, affordable essential medicines and vaccines for all'. If you live in a country with free access to healthcare, it might be difficult to imagine that 30% of the world's population does not have access to essential health services (World Health Organization, 2022). This means people may not have essential medicines, vaccines or treatments.

Practitioner skills activity 2c: Universal health coverage (UHC).

If you were looking at what healthcare services (prevention and treatment) to include in a UHC programme, what do you think you would include? Think of some of the basic things people need in healthcare services and the healthcare needs people have across the life-course.

To provide UHC there needs to be a wide range of policies to support action. For example, healthcare needs to be financed, medicines need to be available and workforces need to be trained. There need to be structures in place that support clean water, sanitation, peace and justice. Ranabhat et al. (2019) suggest that political stability is important for UHC as this ensures funding commitment. Good governance is also important. This means having evaluation and monitoring systems that ensure quality healthcare provision and efficient service delivery. Inequalities continue to restrict access to UHC. Even in counties where healthcare is free, like the UK, some populations such as refugees or migrants or those who are homeless can still find access difficult. See Chapter 5 'Reorientating healthcare services' for more on 'inclusion healthcare'. Examples of innovations in UHC can be found in the wider reading list.

THE HEALTH PROMOTER'S ROLE IN POLICY MAKING

Health promoters can advocate for change by challenging policies that do not support people's rights (see the health promotion in practice examples below about the right to repair and abortion laws) or that negatively impact specific populations. For example, Stonewall campaigns for equality for LGBTQ+ (Lesbian, Gay, Bisexual, Transsexual, Queer and other sexual identities) people including through policy. Their recent work highlights why we should pay attention to the football World Cup in Qatar for LGBTQ+ rights. Read more at https://www.stonewall.org.uk/.

Health promotion in practice example: Abortion rights of women.

Abortion is a medical procedure that ends a pregnancy. Laws that restrict access to this healthcare service impact negatively women and girls. Making abortion illegal does not stop people from ending a pregnancy but makes it less safe to do so. Research by the Economics Observatory (Kobayashi & Thomas, 2022) in the UK (where abortion is legal) suggests differences in abortion service demand. They report younger women living in areas of higher deprivation use abortion services more and therefore unavailability of abortion health services has the biggest impact on poorer, younger women. Globally there is some progress in making abortion legal. The Centre for Reproductive Rights has a map showing country abortion laws at https:// reproductiverights.org/maps/worlds-abortion-laws/.

Health promoters can bring people together with common interests to design and deliver policy action. For example, in areas of the UK community alcohol partnerships (CAP) works with those who sell alcohol, trading standards, the police, health services and education providers to try and reduce underage drinking (this is those under 18 years of age in the UK). Read more at https://www. communityalcoholpartnerships.co.uk/

Health promotion in practice example: The right to repair (EU).

SDG 12 is about 'responsible consumption and production' and many targets reflect the need to reduce waste. The restart project (https:// therestartproject.org/) *helps people to learn to repair their broken electronics. It is also part of the European 'right to repair' campaign. This campaign tries to address the challenge that people face in getting spare parts for electronics so they can be fixed. This makes it difficult to repair, reuse or refurbish items. Remaking and repairing work could reduce waste if people could obtain the correct spare parts. You can read more about the 'right to repair' at* https://repair.eu/.

POLICY CONSULTATION PROCESS

Organisations involved in policymaking may not all share the same views and opinions about action. For example, if a workplace wanted to sell healthy food at a lower cost, catering companies that supply food to the workplace may object. They might suggest adding nutrition information on menus as an alternative. Both can change behaviour, but the cost might influence behaviour more than the provision of information. The consultation process is one way that health promoters can advocate for change. Organisations or people who stand to 'lose' from policies, for example by losing money often have the loudest voices.

Practitioner skills activity 2d: Primary school food provision (UK).

A study that looked at primary school food provision across the UK nations found there is a need for improved school food across the UK (McIntyre et al., 2022). If you were going to create a new school food provision policy in a primary school in your country, who do you think needs to be involved? Would there be any opposition to improving school nutrition standards for example by removing sweets, chocolate or crisps from school snack shops?

In some countries, Governments have 'open' consultations where anyone can comment on policy plans. In Wales, at the time of writing this (2022), current consultations include people affected by suicide and the sale of energy drinks. Some consultations call for evidence which is provided by organisations or groups or interested individuals. For example, the UK Government at the time of writing has a call for evidence for an 'Antimicrobial resistance national action plan'. You can look up the consultations in the UK at England https://www.gov.uk/search/policy-papers-and-consultations, Wales https://gov.wales/consultations, Scotland https://consult.gov.scot/ and Northern Ireland https://www.health-ni.gov.uk/consultations.

Health promotion in practice example: All Party Parliamentary Groups (APPG).

All Party Parliamentary Groups (APPG) promote the interests of specific groups and support members of parliament (MPs) to engage with these issues in the areas they work. The health-related groups differ in content but aim to influence policy-making to improve health. Some group coordinators are well-known organisations. For example, the APPG for dementia is the Alzheimer's Society https://www.alzheimers.org.uk/about-us/policy-and-influencing/all-party-parliamentary-group-dementia *and the APPG for Breast cancer, is Breast Cancer Now* https://breastcancernow.org/get-involved/campaign-us/all-party-parliamentary-group-breast-cancer.

MAKING A HEALTHY POLICY

Making policy is a complex process but most policies follow the same stages. The process is usually represented as a circle although, in reality, policymaking moves between the stages in multiple directions. The main stages are **identification** of the problem, discussion and debate about **solution generation**, **decisions** on what needs to be done, **implementation** and **evaluation** or monitoring of the successes (or failures). Figure 6.5 has an overview of the stages.

IDENTIFYING THE PROBLEM AND SOLUTION GENERATION

As shown in Figure 6.5, policymaking usually starts with the identification of a problem or key issue which has been bought to the attention of those who can make policies. This evidence should tell us things like:

- Whom the problem impacts.
- How serious or likely the problem is.
- The possible outcomes if nothing is done.

Debate and discussion about the problem and the solution uses evidence from a wide range of sources including consultations, benchmarking, public opinion, current local and global affairs and changing trends in mortality and morbidity.

In January 2022 the Department of Transport made changes to 'The Highway Code' to improve the safety of people walking, cycling and riding horses. The Highway Code is the code for all road users in the UK. This process involved a public consultation on The Highway Code Department for Transport (2020). In other policies, issues are bought to the attention through mass media or interested organisations, for example in 2009 there were reported

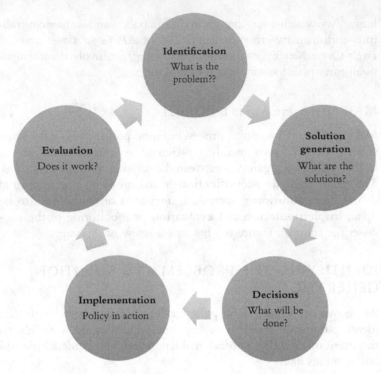

Figure 6.5 Stages of policy making.

links between sunbed use and skin cancer, as well as reports of under-18s using sunbeds in unmanned tanning salons. At the time there was no regulation for sunbed use for those under 18. The Sunbeds (Regulation) Act 2010 which came into force in 2011 prevents those under 18 from using sunbeds based on the evidence accumulated from national and international research (UK Government, 2010). See the health promotion in practice example below about different things to consider in reducing gun violence.

Health promotion in practice example: Preventing gun violence in the United States.

Understanding the causes and risk factors is important in reducing the incidence of gun-based violence in the USA (Sanchez et al., 2020). Rosenberg (2021) suggests four areas that need consideration in policies to reduce gun violence. The first is 'What is the problem?', for example, how many people get shot, who are they and where are they? Secondly, 'what are the causes?', for example, alcohol, poor mental health, poverty and poor housing have all been associated with gun violence, as well as access to guns. Thirdly, 'what works?', for example, what policies and laws can prevent the morbidity and mortality from gun violence, and fourthly, 'how do we do it?', meaning how do we translate and implement these ideas in practice?

DECISION MAKING

Decision-making about policies helps to decide:

- If the population will accept it (acceptability).
- If it is possible to solve the problem with a cost-effective solution (feasibility).
- If it will have the intended effect (effectiveness).
- If there are any other harms or benefits.

One good example is the use of cycle helmets on bicycles. Cycle helmets are not a legal requirement in the UK, although they are mandatory in some countries like Australia. In the UK it has been argued that cycle helmets stop people from cycling, and thus undermine the health benefits of doing the activity. Although evidence suggests helmets can protect the head in an accident, they do not in every scenario and neither do they stop accidents from happening. Organisations like Cycling UK https://www.cyclinguk.org/ and Sustrans https://www.sustrans.org.uk/ state that cycle helmets should be a personal choice and that making people wear them would discourage cycling.

Even when there is good evidence that something will be effective, it does not mean it will happen. It might be very expensive to do, difficult to enforce or strongly opposed. See the example on water fluoridization below.

Health promotion in practice example: Water fluoridization.

In the UK the mineral 'fluoride' occurs naturally in water in varying concentrations. In some areas of England with low natural fluoride levels, fluoride is added to public drinking water. Those areas with fluoride schemes in place have found that water fluoridization is a safe and effective public health measure to reduce dental caries and inequalities in dental health (Office for Health Improvement and Disparities, 2022). Other countries like the USA also actively pursue policies to add fluoride to drinking water to improve dental health (US Department of Health and Human Services, 2023). Some research suggests that high levels of fluoride increase the risk of dental mottling (dental fluorosis). There is unclear and conflicting evidence of the potential harms of fluoride on other areas of health. Consequently, some countries oppose water fluoridization and have no schemes in place.

IMPLEMENTATION AND EVALUATION

'Implementation' is the policy being put into place. Given the need for finance and resources for policy implementation, this process can be slow. Changing social norms is also part of the process. People need to be able to see the benefits of the policy for them. If it is targeting something that is viewed negatively or as socially unacceptable, then people are supportive of the action. Mass media has a role in 'framing' health issues (meaning how they present issues as positive or negative) and influencing what the general public thinks.

Evaluation or monitoring is needed to ensure the policy is effective. The problem may change over time or new evidence might show the problem can be addressed differently. Policies also need to be regularly reviewed for their effect. For example, one way to reduce alcohol consumption is to make alcohol more expensive. Minimum unit pricing (MUP) for alcohol means a unit of alcohol can only be sold at a certain amount (for example in Scotland and Wales this is currently 50p). Research in Australia that analysed wastewater found that MUP reduced consumption in the short term but at 15 months consumption levels increased again (O'Brien et al., 2022). We would want to look at why this might be. It could be aggressive marketing from alcohol companies, an increase in household income, or simply people are used to paying more money for alcohol.

Health promotion in practice example: The food industry (UK).

The food industry, and those who finance it, have a key role to play in changing food environments to make them healthy and sustainable. 'The Food Foundation' says that we need to change the way we produce food and how and what we eat. They argue that food businesses like supermarkets and restaurants should set targets to increase sales of healthy and sustainable foods. 'Peas please: pledge for more veg' is a campaign to increase the UK's vegetable consumption and 'Plating up progress' monitors and scores supermarkets and restaurant chains on areas such as their commitment to improving healthy food sales. Read more at https://foodfoundation.org.uk/. *There is more on food environments and food insecurity in Chapter 4 'Creating supportive environments'.*

HEALTH IMPACT ASSESSMENTS (HIAs)

A Health Impact Assessment (HIA) measures the impact of a policy before it is implemented to see what effect it might have on health. (Ramirez-Rubio et al., 2019) explore a health-in-all-policies approach to improving urban health and supporting countries to achieve the SDGs and recommend the use of HIAs. They suggest that HIAs can help policymakers look at the risks and opportunities through a 'health lens' and information generated by HIA is key in supporting local policies in areas such as active travel, transport and urban greening.

A HIA uses a combination of methods to look at the direct, and indirect effects of what is being proposed on health. For example, traffic calming devices such as speed bumps or speed restrictions in one community can reduce road traffic accidents. However, some vehicles may avoid these areas and take an alternative route through a different community. This can increase the risk of road traffic accidents there instead. A HIA tries to predict these effects. The process is outlined in Figure 6.6.

Figure 6.6 shows the five main stages of the HIA. These are **screening**, where the problem is decided on. **Scoping** where the problem is explored. **Assessing** where you look at whom the policy impacts and how. **Recommendations** are how to reduce the negatives and promote the positives are stated. **Monitoring and evaluation** are when the policy is assessed to check if the HIA predicted the right things.

Practitioner skills activity 2e: Policy stakeholders.

SDG 5 aims to achieve gender equality and empower all women and girls. A coalition of local organisations has planned a policy to eliminate all forms of violence against women and girls in public and private spaces (SDG indicator 5.2). The

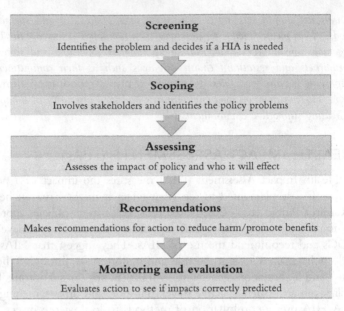

Figure 6.6 The health impact assessment process.

project intends to work with everyone in the community to a) encourage reporting of interpersonal violence (IPV) to authorities and healthcare workers and b) improve the environments where women and girls report feeling unsafe. What stakeholders do you think will need to be involved with this project? What might be the positive and negative impacts of this project? Can you see any potential harm from this project?

The HIA process starts by identifying relevant stakeholders (meaning people who have a 'stake' or an interest in the policy in some way). This could be voluntary groups, businesses or the general public. Stakeholders identify the positive and negative impacts of the policy including the impact on vulnerable populations. They also look at barriers to putting a policy in place and possible solutions. There is a wide range of tools that can support the HIA process. One example is HEAT for walking and cycling by the WHO (World Health Organization, 2021). This is an online tool that helps people to calculate the health impacts and economic benefits of walking or cycling. You can read more about HEAT at https://www.heatwalkingcycling.org/. The Institute of Public Health in Northern Ireland has a HIA manual, case studies and videos about Health Impact Assessments at https://publichealth.ie/hia-guidance/. The Welsh Institute of Health Impact Assessments also has a wide range of case studies at https://phwwhocc.co.uk/whiasu/. There is also an example below.

Health promotion in practice example: HIAs in East and West Africa.

Large-scale infrastructure projects like mining can cause environmental or geographical changes to communities that can impact health. Many African countries have valuable minerals like gold and copper which need to be extracted from underground. The negative impact of mining on environments and ecosystems is known but what is less clear is how mining projects impact the wider determinants of health in local communities. Leuenberger et al. (2022) explore HIAs in four East and West African countries (Mozambique, Tanzania, Ghana and Burkina Faso) as part of a larger research initiative 'Health Impact Assessment for Sustainable Development' (HIA4SD). They show how HIAs can be used in ways that are more participatory and represent the views of different groups of people. The article provides a practical toolbox of resources for people working in these areas. The toolbox suggests non-traditional ways of collecting data such as 'a transect walk'. This is a walk through an area guided by local informants. The toolkits are available through the journal article (see reference list at end). You can also read more about HIA4SD at https://hia4sd.net/.

DIFFERENT POLICIES FOR DIFFERENT PURPOSES

In many countries, Governments still create policies that promote individual behaviour change rather than structural or environmental change. Research suggests that policies that focus on individual change have been found to increase inequalities. This is because those who can change their behaviour are more likely to have the resources, time, money or skills to do so. For example, Coupe et al. (2018) note that changes in Government policies to address unhealthy behaviours in the UK have resulted in improvements for those in higher socio-economic groups, but not those in lower socio-economic groups. An example in Bradford (England) identifies that around 10% of annual premature deaths could be prevented if there was compliance with the recommended levels for physical activity, air and noise pollution and green space access (Mueller et al., 2018). These areas require policy changes or stricter enforcement of existing regulations. Residents in lower-income neighbourhoods have the highest risk and recommendations include interventions that prioritise these areas as this is where the largest gains are to be had.

Policies that focus on changing the conditions where people live have more potential to reduce inequalities. This means having different policies for the same aim. See the health promotion practice example below about 'policy packages'. A recent successful example is the soft drinks industry levy or 'sugar tax'. This law requires manufacturers to pay a tax on the sugar amount in their products. The idea is that companies that make foods or drinks with sugar either regulate and reduce the sugar they use or pay the levy. You can read more about countries that have a 'sugar tax' in the 'food environment' section of Chapter 4 'Creating supportive environments'.

Health promotion in practice example: Policy packages for diet and physical activity (EU).

The Organisation for Economic Co-operation and Development (OECD) is an international organisation that works to build better policies. A report 'Healthy eating and active lifestyles' found most OECD countries have action plans for an unhealthy diet and physical activity. These plans show four main policy areas. They try to influence people to make healthier choices (like food labelling), widen the availability of choices (like green space access), change prices of unhealthy products (adding tax), or restrict access to unhealthy foods (banning foods). The report recommends that countries use different policies to change behaviours and environments and that policies target the needs of disadvantaged groups. Read more at https://www.oecd.org/health/.

THE INTERVENTION LADDER

The Nuffield Council on Bioethics (The Nuffield Council on Bioethics, 2007) uses an intervention ladder as a way of thinking about

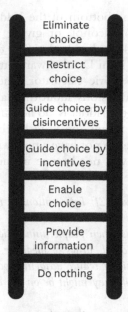

Figure 6.7 The Nuffield Council of Bioethics Intervention ladder.

the different ways that health policies impact people's choices. A policy is not just in place to ban things that might be bad for health. Policies can be used in many different ways to support health. Figure 6.7 shows the intervention ladder and the different policy levels.

As Figure 6.7 shows, policies at the top of the ladder stop people from doing things. They need a strong reason for their use. An example is the ban on driving under the influence of alcohol (drink driving). Evidence suggests drink driving is associated with significant harm and that enforcing legislation to reduce it works (Anderson et al., 2009). In the UK, drink driving is subject to harsh laws that punish offenders with penalties such as large fines and driving bans.

Policies in the middle of the ladder include Age ID schemes for buying alcohol or specific licensing hours which say when a business can sell alcohol. These both restrict access to alcohol to protect people but alcohol can still be drunk.

Policies closer to the bottom of the ladder include health education on the risks of alcohol, or giving information about the calories or units in alcoholic drinks. See for example the health information resources from Drink Aware https://www.drinkaware.co.uk/tools/unit-and-calorie-calculator. These policies give people information to make decisions about their alcohol use.

The lowest layer of the ladder is 'do nothing'. This does not mean ignoring the issue. It means the issue has been looked at and has been decided it is better to not have a policy in place at present. This does not mean there will not be one in the future. See the water fluoridization example above.

Practitioner skills activity 2f: Interventions to reduce accidental poisoning in young people.

Accidental poisoning is when people unintentionally harm themselves by taking something like alcohol, drugs or medicine. Look at the list of interventions that can potentially reduce accidental poisoning in children under five. Where do you think they might be on the ladder in Figure 6.6?

- *Restrictions on how many packets of non-prescription painkillers you can purchase in supermarkets.*
- *Compulsory manufacturer safety caps on all medicines.*
- *Telling parents or carers to not store medicines or chemicals near food.*
- *A local pharmacy scheme where people can hand back medication that is not needed.*
- *Schools-based education for young people.*

TACKLING ILLEGAL DRUG USE THROUGH POLICIES

SDG indicator 3.5 focuses on strengthening the prevention and treatment of substance abuse. In many countries, drugs are illegal unless they have been prescribed for medical reasons. However, they are still taken by some people and consequently, this may result in harm. This is called 'substance abuse'. In the UK, drugs that cause major harm such as Heroin and Cocaine are illegal. You can read more about different types of drugs at 'Talktofrank'

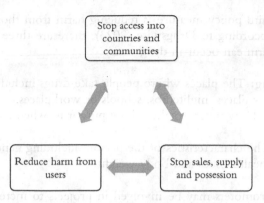

Figure 6.8 Three main policy approaches to illegal drugs.

https://www.talktofrank.com/. The main policy approaches to tackling illegal drugs are shown in Figure 6.8.

Figure 6.8 shows the three main policy approaches. These are:

• Reducing access to drugs by stopping them from entering the country or halting their movement of them across the country.
• Prosecuting those who sell or have drugs.
• Reducing harm from those who use drugs.

The first two policy approaches are connected. Reducing access to drugs involves policies to stop drugs from entering a country or from reaching users. In the UK most illegal drugs come from outside the UK and therefore have to be imported into the country. Border and customs control and restricting the movement of drugs across 'county lines' are the main policy responses. 'County lines' is a term that refers to the organised movement of drugs from cities to towns via a network of people. Prosecution includes anyone who takes drugs, carries drugs, makes drugs or sells drugs. This can be a prison sentence or a fine depending on the class of the drug. In the UK large organisations like the National Crime Agency https://nationalcrimeagency.gov.uk/ and local police forces are involved in reducing access to drugs and trying to stop those who sell drugs.

The third policy measure is reducing harm from those who use drugs. According to Drugswise (2023), there are three main areas where harm can occur in drug users.

- **Setting:** The places where people take drugs including out-of-the-way places, nightclubs, schools or workplaces.
- **Drug:** How much is taken, how pure it is, when and how it is taken.
- **Set:** The characteristics of the person, including gender, underlying health issues and body weight.

Health promoters may be involved in projects to increase knowledge of drugs and reduce harm from drug taking. These can focus on any or all of the three areas (setting, drug, set). Interventions include the provision of needle exchange programmes or safe injecting sites focusing on the 'setting' where drugs are taken to reduce risks and harms. Schools-based or university-based drug education aimed at increasing knowledge of drugs, or drug testing at festivals is aimed at the 'drug'. Identifying individual risks and tailoring interventions such as drug use in pregnancy, or knowledge about how drugs impact people differently, focuses on 'set'.

Drug services for those looking to reduce or stop drugs are part of a strong policy environment. The provision of drug addiction services and supervised opioid withdrawal treatment to reduce harm from drugs are essential, as those taking drugs may need considerable support to stop. Chapter 2 'Developing personal skills' has an example of a 'Naxolone' intervention used to prevent drug overdose. For more on different types of interventions see the Drugswise encyclopaedia at https://www.drugwise.org.uk/drugsearch-encyclopedia/ and for factsheets see https://www.drugwise.org.uk/factsheets-and-infographics/.

TACKLING CLIMATE CHANGE THROUGH POLICIES

Climate change threatens human health and well-being. The Paris Agreement is a United Nations 'pact' that 195 states have signed. The purpose of the agreement is to limit climate change and strengthen the global response. There are three purposes; to limit temperature changes to 1.5°C, to review country commitments to reducing climate change every five years, and to provide climate change finance to low-income countries. You can read more about The Paris Agreement at https://www.un.org/en/climatechange/paris-agreement.

The Lancet Countdown on health and climate change publishes a yearly report on health and climate. Their most recent countdown report can be found here https://www.thelancet.com/countdown-health-climate. The report tells us about the impact of climate change on health. As temperatures get higher and weather patterns change, this impacts humans in different ways. For example, it can cause drought, and food insecurity, and increase the risk of diseases like Malaria (transmitted by mosquitos). Extreme weather such as floods and droughts impacts people, livelihoods and living conditions, and those who are most vulnerable experience these effects the most.

Doing something about climate change requires action from everyone. Policies need to involve all sectors of society from individuals to Governments and across areas like textiles and clothing, food and drinks, electronics and technology, manufacturing and construction.

Practitioner skills activity 2f: Reaching Net Zero.

Some countries have committed to reaching Net Zero. There are videos about what is NetZero at the UN Net Zero coalition website at https://www.un.org/en/climatechange/net-zero-coalition. You can also track your country's progress to achieving the SDGs that are connected to climate change, for example, SDG 12: Responsible consumption and production and SDG 13: Climate action. Use the SDG dashboard https://dashboards.sdgindex.org/profiles.

There are two main types of policy in climate change.

- Mitigation policies are strategies that tackle the causes of climate change.
- Adaptation policies to reduce the negative impacts of climate change.

Mitigation and adaptation policies are shown with examples in Figure 6.9. The explanation of these areas is below:

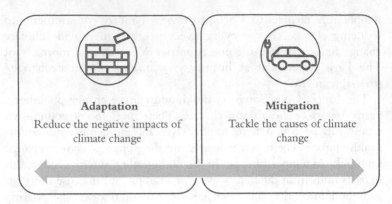

Figure 6.9 Adaptation and mitigation for climate change.

Mitigation policies focus on areas like making buildings more energy efficient and reducing fossil fuel consumption. This means burning less coal, oil and gas and finding different ways to provide energy. Changing cars and lorries from petrol to electric and using cleaner energy such as solar power or wind power are two examples. Carbon Tax is a policy that makes people pay a fee for burning fossil fuels. It makes organisations that pollute the most pay money which can be invested in other solutions like alternative energy sources.

Adaptation policies recognise that climate change is happening. They try and make things safer or stronger so they are better able to deal with rising temperatures or more extreme weather. This could be building safer climate-proof buildings or structures like bridges, planting or replanting trees, diversifying crops to include drought-resistant crops and having robust emergency plans in place for heatwaves or flooding.

PROMOTING ACTIVE TRAVEL THROUGH POLICIES

In the UK local authorities are responsible for local transport plans. Good planning and regulations can reduce preventable deaths and injuries by reducing pollution, promoting active travel and connecting communities. There are substantial health gains and healthcare cost savings from switching short car trips to walking and cycling, as well as reductions in carbon emissions from vehicles (Mizdrak et al., 2019). Policies that focus on promoting public transport and active travel have the most benefits to offer and can reduce health inequalities. You can read more about transport and health using The Health Foundation resource https://www.health. org.uk/infographic/transport-and-health.

'Gear change: A bold vision for cycling and walking' (Department for Transport, 2020) is a policy document that aspires to make England a great walking and cycling nation. The policy states that active travel can reduce congestion, promote local businesses, contribute to the economy and improve the environment and air quality.

The plan has four themes:

(1)   Better streets for cycling and people.
(2)   Cycling and walking at the heart of decision-making.
(3)   Empowering and encouraging local authorities.
(4)   Enabling people to cycle and protecting them when they do.

Each theme has 'design principles'. For example, theme 1 'better streets for cycling and people' states that cycle routes must be designed for large numbers of cyclists and different abilities and disabilities. This includes separating cyclists from pedestrians and vehicles, making sure routes are well marked, taking account of how cyclists behave, and being designed by people who have experienced roads on a bicycle.

Health promotion in practice example: Station travel plans in Scotland.

ScotRail publishes station travel plans for several Scottish train stations. Station travel plans are a tool to help promote connectivity between communities and railway stations. They explore the different ways that stations can promote access and encourage sustainable ways to get to and from a railway station. For example, Bathgate station (Glasgow) shows problems with parking congestion, people making short car trips to the station, and a lack of reliable assistance or facilities. They also explore the 'last mile' (a term used for how people get from the station to their home) and found no cycle lanes and a lack of pedestrian crossings. The action plan states several actions, including that the station will promote and integrate with local bus services and reduce parking congestion through a modal shift. This means people moving from one form of transport to another such as a car to bike. For

Scottish station travel plans see https://www.scotrail.co.uk/plan-your-journey/travel-connections/station-travel-plans.

REDUCING TEENAGE PREGNANCY THROUGH POLICIES

Globally, reducing pregnancy in adolescents 15–19 is essential to achieving the SDGs related to maternal and newborn health as adolescents often have a higher risk of poor maternal health outcomes. Maternal conditions are among the top causes of disability-adjusted life years (DALYs) and death among girls aged 15–19 (UNICEF, 2023). There are health consequences associated with not just birth in adolescence, but also the spacing between subsequent births, and the total number of births to each adolescent mother. These can bring consequences to the physical, social and psychological health and well-being of young mothers and their children.

Adolescent birth is influenced by a range of factors. These are shown in Figure 6.10.

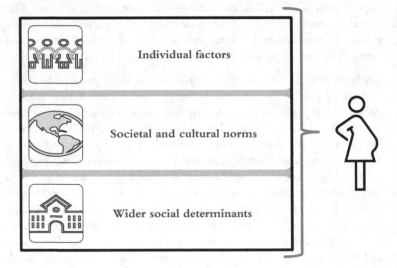

Figure 6.10 Factors that influence the adolescent birth rate.

Figure 6.10 shows the three main factors that influence the adolescent birth rate. They include:

- **Individual factors** such as sexual debut and frequency of sexual activity.
- **Societal and cultural norms** such as the value of women, patterns of marriage and access and acceptability of contraception.
- **Wider societal determinants** such as education for girls, employment prospects, peace, political commitment and economic development.

Although some young people choose to have a child before the age of 18, many young people do not. In the UK, research shows that mothers aged under 18 are more likely to drop out of education, live in poverty and have a higher risk of mental health problems than older mothers (Nuffield Trust, 2023). Young women may be forced to leave school, which impacts their education and employment opportunities and their ability to earn money. There are also social consequences such as stigma, or rejection by family, partners, or friends.

In the UK, whilst under-18 conceptions have been decreasing in the UK (Office of National Statistics, 2022) many other countries are making better progress at decreasing teenage pregnancy across Europe including the Netherlands and Denmark (Office of National Statistics, 2018). 'The Teenage pregnancy prevention Framework' (Public Health England, 2018) is a way England has set out ways to try and reduce teenage pregnancy. The framework sets out ten areas that different agencies should focus on underpinned by two core concepts; leadership and accountability. The framework states that strategic leadership is essential to reducing teenage pregnancy, and accountability for services, delivery and commissioning (meaning buying health services to reflect local needs) is also needed. The ten core areas include relationships and sex education in schools, targeted prevention for young people most at risk, advice and access to contraception in non-health education and youth settings, and youth friendly sexual health services.

Different countries' approaches to teenage pregnancy policies share similar values of leadership and accountability underpinning their strategies. For example in Ghana, the five-year strategic plan to reduce adolescent pregnancy (Ministry of gender children and social protection, 2017) includes a focus on organisational development, institutional governance, resource mobilisation and capacity building. All elements are needed for a strong policy.

Health promotion in practice example: Thailand's Act to prevent adolescent pregnancy.

In 2016 Thailand introduced the 'Act for Prevention and solution of the adolescent pregnancy problem' (Government of Thailand, 2016). This law tries to coordinate efforts to target teenage pregnancy. It has key measures to provide support via schools, workplaces, public health facilities, social welfare organisations and local administrative organisations. It includes the provision of age-appropriate sexuality education, access to reproductive services and promoting adolescent rights. More recently the Act has been amended to stop educational institutions from expelling or transferring pregnant students from schools and to provide maternity leave to young mothers in schools. You can watch a video about the Act at https://www.youtube.com/watch?v=uHnZgphvzIw *and see mass media resources at* https://thailand.unfpa.org/en/node/15684.

To read more on global adolescent pregnancy see the United Nations Population Fund section on Adolescents which includes a range of data at https://www.unfpa.org/adolescent-pregnancy. A resource 'Motherhood in Childhood: The Untold Story (United Nations Population Fund, 2022) has also been produced to tell the stories of young mothers at https://www.unfpa.org/publications/motherhood-childhood-untold-story.

Practitioner skills activity 2g: Reproductive rights, laws and policies.

Explore one of the United Nations Population Fund countries to see what rights, laws and policies it has in place to support reproductive rights. Choose a country and this link https://www.unfpa.org/data *and explore the 'key results' sections (and the news section). If you are not sure which country to look at here are some links to five different countries: Bangladesh* https://www.unfpa.org/data/BD, *Libya* https://www.unfpa.org/data/LY, *Nigeria* https://www.unfpa.org/data/NG, *Brazil* https://www.unfpa.org/data/BR *and Ukraine* https://www.unfpa.org/data/UA.

CHALLENGES TO HEALTHY PUBLIC POLICY

There are multiple challenges to creating healthy public policy. One of the biggest is that the concentration of wealth and power often rests with those who have the most to lose. This is often represented as a 'conflict of interest'. Taxes on products such as tobacco, alcohol, high fat and high sugar foods face significant opposition from the companies that make these products and the power and influence they have. Political commitment is also difficult. Some Governments may only be in power for four or five years, making long-term plans difficult.

One policy by itself is a good starting point, but it might not be enough to make big changes that are needed across society. Multiple policies are usually needed. Strong policies need the resources to be effective, such as finance, political will, good governance and enforcement so the policy does what it intends to do.

SUMMARY

Healthy public policy is perhaps one of the most challenging areas of health promotion, especially when health promoters have no way of being part of the policy agenda in health. Policymaking can also be a slow process that takes many years to show any result. However, as global issues like climate change, Covid-19 and the Russian-Ukraine conflict have shown us, health is global and what happens in one country will have an impact on another. Health promoters need to actively campaign for changes to policies that damage health to protect population health locally, nationally and internationally. They need to be part of policy consultations and use their skills to show others how policy has the potential to improve health now and in future generations.

WIDER READING

ONLINE

Policy changes so it is recommended that you keep up to date with your own country's health policies through their Government websites. Health Policy Watch has global policy stories and health news at https://healthpolicy-watch.news/.

Active Neighbourhoods Canada (2023). Co-designing the health city healthy public policy toolkit (Canada-based). https://participatoryplanning.ca/.

The Health Foundation (2019). Implementing health in all policies: Lessons from around the world. Available at https://www.health.org.uk/publications.

The Lancet series for example Public Health Systems https://www.thelancet.com/series/public-health-systems Road safety https://www.thelancet.com/series/road-safety Trade and health, https://www.thelancet.com/series/trade-and-health, Tobacco free world Tobacco-free world (thelancet.com).

The Lancet series on UHC: Bangladesh: Innovation for Universal Health Coverage, https://www.thelancet.com/series/bangladesh, Universal Health care coverage in Latin America, https://www.thelancet.com/series/latin-america-UHC.

The World Bank (2023). The world by income and region at https://datatopics.worldbank.org/world-development-indicators/the-world-by-income-and-region.html.

United Nations Population Fund has many resources for countries including their current policies and health promotion programmes as well as data. Data can be found at https://www.unfpa.org/data.

TEXTBOOKS

This book looks at different countries. Blank, R. H., Burau, V., & Khulmann, E. (2017). *Comparative health policy*. 5th Edition. Palgrave Macmillan, Basingstoke.

Buse, K., Mays, N., & Walt, G. (2013). *Making health policy*. 2nd ed. McGraw-Hill/Open University Press, Maidenhead.

Hunter, D. J. (2003). *Public health policy*. Polity Press, Cambridge.

LISTENING AND WATCHING

The Kings Fund Podcasts 'What just happened. Health and care policy in 2021', and 'Charting the Nation's Health' with John Burn-Murdoch' both available from The Kings Fund website https://www.kingsfund.org.uk/ or your podcast provider.

American Public Health Association. What does "health in all policies" mean? Episode 9 of "That's Public Health" available at What does "health in all policies" mean? Episode 9 of "That's Public Health" - YouTube.

Crash course (US-based) video shorts on: How Laws Affect Your Health: Crash Course Public Health #8 available at https://www.youtube.com/watch?v=Z08sh4PN8Lc. How the Environment Affects Your Health: Crash Course Public Health #3 https://www.youtube.com/watch?v=g3vf0I_j9kk, How Society Affects Your Health: Crash Course Public Health #4 https://www.youtube.com/watch?v=CcdSeqqMR5M Which Healthcare System is Best? Crash Course Public Health #7 https://www.youtube.com/watch?v=vxvhGj9fA3g.

ADDITIONAL REFERENCES

These are the additional references this chapter has used where electronic links have not been provided in the chapter.

Anderson, P., Chisholm, D., & Fuhr, D. C. (2009). Effectiveness and cost-effectiveness of policies and programmes to reduce the harm caused by alcohol. *Lancet*, *373*(9682), 2234–2246. 10.1016/s0140-6736(09)60744-3.

Coupe, N., Cotterill, S., & Peters, S. (2018). Tailoring lifestyle interventions to low socio-economic populations: a qualitative study. *BMC Public Health*, *18*(1), 967. 10.1186/s12889-018-5877-8.

Department for Transport. (2020). Gear change: a bold vision for cycling and walking. Available at https://www.gov.uk/government/publications/cycling-and-walking-plan-for-england.

Department of Health. (2014). Making life better: Strategic framework for public health. Available at https://www.health-ni.gov.uk/articles/making-life-better-strategic-framework-public-health.

Drugswise. (2023). What are the dangers from using drugs. Available at https://www.drugwise.org.uk/wp-content/uploads/What-are-the-dangers-fro-using-drugs.png.

European Commission. (2023). #EUSPI The EU Social Progress Index 2020. Available at https://cohesiondata.ec.europa.eu/stories/s/EU-Social-Progress-Index-2020/8qk9-xq96.

Government of Thailand. (2016). Act for prevention and solution of the adolescent pregnancy problem. Available at http://web.krisdika.go.th/data/document/ext810/810252_0001.pdf.

Jiang, B., Liang, S., Peng, Z. R., Cong, H., Levy, M., Cheng, Q., Wang, T., & Remais, J. V. (2017). Transport and public health in China: The road to a healthy future. *Lancet*, *390*(10104), 1781–1791. 10.1016/s0140-6736(17)31958-x.

Kabir, H., Maple, M., Usher, K., & Islam, M. S. (2019). Health vulnerabilities of readymade garment (RMG) workers: a systematic review. *BMC Public Health*, *19*(1), 70. 10.1186/s12889-019-6388-y.

Kobayashi, A., & Thomas, M. (2022). Does access to abortion vary across the UK. Economics Observatory. Available at https://www.economicsobservatory.com/does-access-to-abortion-vary-across-the-uk.

Leuenberger, A., Winkler, M. S., Lyatuu, I., Cossa, H., Zabré, H. R., Dietler, D., & Farnham, A. (2022). Incorporating community perspectives in health impact assessment: A toolbox. *Environmental Impact Assessment Review*, *95*, 106788. 10.1016/j.eiar.2022.106788.

McIntyre, R. L., Adamson, A. J., Nelson, M., Woodside, J., Beattie, S., & Spence, S. (2022). Changes and differences in school food standards (2010-2021) and free school meal provision during COVID-19 across the UK: Potential implications for children's diets. *Nutr Bull, 47*(2), 230–245. 10.1111/nbu.12556.

Ministry of gender children and social protection. (2017). Five year strategic plan to address adolescent pregnancy in Ghana 2018-2022. Available at https://ghana.unfpa.org/sites/default/files/pub-pdf/Adolescent%20Pregnancy%20Strategic%20Plan%202018.pdf.

Mizdrak, A., Blakely, T., Cleghorn, C. L., & Cobiac, L. J. (2019). Potential of active transport to improve health, reduce healthcare costs, and reduce greenhouse gas emissions: A modelling study. *PLoS One, 14*(7), e0219316. 10.1371/journal.pone.0219316.

Mueller, N., Rojas-Rueda, D., Khreis, H., Cirach, M., Milà, C., Espinosa, A., Foraster, M., McEachan, R. R. C., Kelly, B., Wright, J., & Nieuwenhuijsen, M. (2018). Socioeconomic inequalities in urban and transport planning related exposures and mortality: A health impact assessment study for Bradford, UK. *Environment International, 121*, 931–941. 10.1016/j.envint.2018.10.017.

New Zealand Government. (2022). Budget 2022: The wellbeing outlook and approach. Available at https://budget.govt.nz/budget/2022/wellbeing/outlook/index.htm.

Nuffield Trust. (2023). Teenage pregnancy. Available at https://www.nuffieldtrust.org.uk/resource/teenage-pregnancy.

O'Brien, J. W., Tscharke, B. J., Bade, R., Chan, G., Gerber, C., Mueller, J. F., Thomas, K. V., & Hall, W. D. (2022). A wastewater-based assessment of the impact of a minimum unit price (MUP) on population alcohol consumption in the Northern Territory, Australia. *Addiction, 117*(1), 243–249. 10.1111/add.15631.

Office for Health Improvement and Disparities. (2022). Water fluoridation: Health monitoring report for England 2022. Available at https://assets.publishing.service.gov.uk/government/uploads/system/uploads/attachment_data/file/1060471/water-fluoridation-health-monitoring-report-2022.pdf.

Office of National Statistics. (2018). Live birth rates to women aged under 18 and under 20 years, in EU28 countries, 2006, 2015 and 2016. Available at https://www.ons.gov.uk/peoplepopulationandcommunity/birthsdeathsandmarriages/livebirths/adhocs/008261livebirthratestowomenagedunder18andunder20yearsineu28countries20062015and2016.

Office of National Statistics. (2022). Conceptions in England and Wales 2020. Available at https://www.ons.gov.uk/peoplepopulationandcommunity/birthsdeathsandmarriages/conceptionandfertilityrates/bulletins/conceptionstatistics/2020.

Public Health England. (2018). Teenage pregnancy prevention framework. Available at https://www.gov.uk/government/publications/teenage-pregnancy-prevention-framework.

Public Health England. (2019). Public Health strategy 2020-2025. Available at https://www.gov.uk/government/publications/phe-strategy-2020-to-2025.

Public Health Wales. (2018). Working to achieve a healthier future for Wales: Long term strategy 2018-2030. Available at https://phw.nhs.wales/about-us/our-priorities/.

Ramirez-Rubio, O., Daher, C., Fanjul, G., Gascon, M., Mueller, N., Pajín, L., Plasencia, A., Rojas-Rueda, D., Thondoo, M., & Nieuwenhuijsen, M. J. (2019). Urban health: An example of a "health in all policies" approach in the context of SDGs implementation. *Globalization and Health, 15*(1), 87. 10.1186/s12992-019-0529-z.

Ranabhat, C. L., Jakovljevic, M., Dhimal, M., & Kim, C. B. (2019). Structural factors responsible for universal health coverage in low- and middle-income countries: Results from 118 countries. *Frontiers in Public Health, 7*, 414. 10.33 89/fpubh.2019.00414.

Rosenberg, M. (2021). Considerations for developing an agenda for gun violence prevention research. *Annual Review in Public Health, 42*, 23–41. 10.114 6/annurev-publhealth-012420-105117.

Sanchez, C., Jaguan, D., Shaikh, S., McKenney, M., & Elkbuli, A. (2020). A systematic review of the causes and prevention strategies in reducing gun violence in the United States. *American Journal of Emergency Medicine, 38*(10), 2169–2178. 10.1016/j.ajem.2020.06.062.

Scottish Government. (2018). Scotland's Public Health Priorities. Available at https://www.gov.scot/publications/scotlands-public-health-priorities/pages/1/.

The Nuffield Council on Bioethics. (2007). The intervention ladder. Available at https://www.nuffieldbioethics.org/publications/public-health/guide-to-the-report/policy-process-and-practice.

The Samaritans. (2023). Campaign for a suicide-safer internet. Available at https://www.samaritans.org/wales/about-samaritans/research-policy/internet-suicide/campaign-safer-internet/.

UK Government. (2010). Sunbeds (Regulations) Act 2010: Guidance on the implementation of the Sunbeds (Regulation) Act 2010. Available at https://www.gov.uk/government/publications/sunbeds-regulations-act-2010-guidance-on-the-implementation-of-the-sunbeds-regulation-act-2010.

UK Government. (2022). Smoking at work. The law. Available at https://www.gov.uk/smoking-at-work-the-law.

UNICEF. (2023). Early childbearing. Available at https://data.unicef.org/topic/child-health/adolescent-health/.

United Nations Population Fund. (2022). Motherhood in childhood: The untold story. Available at https://www.unfpa.org/publications/motherhood-childhood-untold-story.

US Department of Health and Human Services. (2023). Increase the proportion of people whose water systems have the recommended amount of fluoride objective. Available at https://health.gov/healthypeople/objectives-and-data/browse-objectives/health-policy/increase-proportion-people-whose-water-systems-have-recommended-amount-fluoride-oh-11.

Welsh Government. (2015). Wellbeing for Future Generations Act. Available at https://www.futuregenerations.wales/about-us/future-generations-act/.

World Health Organization. (1986). The Ottawa charter for health promotion: First international conference on health promotion, Ottawa, 21 November 1986. Available at https://www.who.int/teams/health-promotion/enhanced-wellbeing/first-global-conference.

World Health Organization. (2021). Health economic assessment tool (HEAT) for walking and cycling by WHO. Available at https://www.heatwalkingcycling.org/.

World Health Organization. (2022). Universal Health Coverage. Available at https://www.who.int/health-topics/universal-health-coverage#tab=tab_1.

World Health Organization. (2023). Banning tobacco advertising, sponsorship and promotion. Available at https://www.who.int/europe/health-topics/tobacco/banning-tobacco-advertising-sponsorship-and-promotion#tab=tab_1.

LAST WORDS, FIRST ACTIONS

We need creative, innovative and original thinking to achieve health for all. Poverty, inequality and inequity can only be reduced with new ways of working. Tackling climate change, the increasing burden of communicable diseases and new diseases that cross global borders are long-term challenges. If the Covid-19 outbreak gave us one thing, it was the opportunity to try different problem-solving approaches. It has shown us how health services can rapidly change the way they are delivered. Changes that might normally have taken years were achieved in weeks, and technology was used in ways that previously were not considered possible. This change is not just seen in healthcare, but in education, workplaces and in the communities where we live.

This book has shown you the many ways to advocate, enable and mediate change in health promotion using the five action areas of the Ottawa Charter. It has given you examples of how others are working to create change and support the health of future generations. Now it is your turn. Reflect on what you have been learning in this book, and what topics and activities you are most interested in, or feel really passionate about. You are the future of health promotion, and the health of individuals, communities and countries is in your hands.

What will you do next?

DOI: 10.4324/9781003462323-8

GLOSSARY

Behaviour change When people change what they do to try and be healthier such as eating a different diet or taking more physical activity.

Behaviour change theory or model A theory or model that is used to try and predict how people change their behaviour. It usually has variables like attitude, knowledge or motivation.

Bottom-up and top down Messages or programmes designed by healthcare practitioners to be delivered to a target group without involving the target group come from the 'top', meaning top-down. Those designed using the experiences, words and knowledge of the target group come from the bottom, so bottom-up. Sometimes we also call bottom-up 'user-led'.

Campaign, initiative, intervention or programme Mass media health communication is usually in the form of a campaign. Initiatives, interventions or programmes are similar but usually refer to a project of some sort that aims to try and improve health and may or may not use media.

Climate change The increasing changes in climate and temperature through the burning of fossil fuels. When we burn fossil fuels like coal or oil, the emissions act like a 'greenhouse', and trap the heat closer to the Earth. This is the 'greenhouse effect'. This raises temperatures. Climate change has major consequences for our health. Read more at https://www.un.org/en/climatechange/what-is-climate-change

Communicable disease Infectious diseases like HIV, Tuberculosis, measles or influenza.

Governance People who are in charge and make decisions about services including policies are accountable or responsible for actions. Good governance tries to ensure services are good quality, safe, inclusive, meet demand and are well resourced.

Cultural safety Being culturally aware and ensuring healthcare practice is respectful, non-discriminatory, inclusive and listens to the needs of those who are different to ourselves.

Covid-19 (coronavirus) SARS-cov-2 is viral respiratory disease passed from person to person. Most people have a mild or moderate illness and do not need treatment. The virus was first reported in December 2019. Before a vaccine, many countries were 'locked down'. People were not allowed out of their homes except for essential reasons. The first vaccines were given towards the end of 2021.

Department of Health/Ministry of Health This is the Government department with responsibility for health in a country.

Deprivation Not having certain resources or assets that are essential to life like decent housing or safe streets. Those people who are in a lower socio-economic status often live in areas of high deprivation (see 'socioeconomic status' below).

Health communication The design and delivery of health messages across different channels such as face to face and mass media.

Health inequalities The unequal differences between people and their health. This can be seen in areas like life expectancy, access to quality housing, decent work or healthcare services.

Health inequities The unfair differences between people and their health. This is the failure to recognise that some people need more support than others to be 'equal'.

Health literacy The ability to locate, understand and apply health information.

Health promotion A discipline that advocates, enables and mediates change to promote good health and prevent ill health in individuals, communities and wider society.

Health protection An area of public health that protects populations from hazards and risks such as infectious disease, violence or climate-related weather events such as floods.

Health psychology A discipline that uses psychological science to explore behaviours in health and illness.

Healthy life expectancy The number of years someone is expected to live in good health.

Healthy lifestyles When people adopt behaviours in their lifestyle such as stopping smoking or cutting down on their alcohol to be healthier.

Information Technology (IT) Includes the internet, social media platforms and mobile phones and their apps. It also includes wearable technology such as smart watches.

LGBTQ That means Lesbian, Gay, Bisexual, Transexual, Queer and other sexual identities.

Life expectancy The number of years someone is expected to live.

Mass media Includes posters, leaflets, billboards, radio, television, newspapers or other audio-visual communication used to promote health.

National Health Service (NHS) The UK's health service that offers free universal healthcare at point of access. It is mainly paid for by taxation and National Insurance contributions.

Non-communicable disease Non-infectious diseases or 'chronic' diseases like cancer, stroke, cardiovascular disease or diabetes.

Prevention Stopping something before it happens such as the risk of a disease.

Public health The 'science' of protecting health that aims to reduce threats to population health and usually includes health protection, epidemiology and surveillance. Sometimes health promotion is included under the umbrella of public health.

Social capital The social resources that someone has such as their family, friends or community networks.

Social determinants of health The factors around us that influence our health such as access to decent and secure housing, employment, education or income.

Socioeconomic status Our supposed status in society based on our occupation. Those with higher paid jobs with more responsibilities usually have a higher socio-economic status. Those who are unemployed or working in lower paid work have usually lower socio-economic status. This is sometimes used as a way to explore health inequalities as those with higher socio-economic status generally have better health and better access to services or resources.

Sustainable development goal (SDGs) Seventeen global goals (including 169 targets) for peace, prosperity and health across the world to be achieved by 2030. United Nations member states adopted the goals in 2015, for achievement by 2030. Read more at https://sdgs.un.org/

Universal Health Coverage (UHC) Means people have access to healthcare services when they need them without experience financial problems obtaining them. The NHS is one example (see 'National Health service' above).

United Kingdom (four nations) The United Kingdom is made up of four countries: England, Northern Ireland, Scotland and Wales. It is situated in Europe.

World Health Organization (WHO) Global organisation that leads and supports efforts to achieve better health for all https://www.who.int/

INDEX